SECOND EDITION

The Health Care Data Source Book

Finding the right information and making the most of it

John D. Fry
Diana B. McKinnie
Robert W. Young

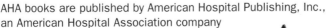
AHA books are published by American Hospital Publishing, Inc.,
an American Hospital Association company

Library of Congress Cataloging-in-Publication Data

Fry, John D.
   The health care data source book : finding the right information and making the most of it / John D. Fry, Diana B. McKinnie, Robert W. Young.—2nd ed.
        p.   cm.
   Includes bibliographical references.
   ISBN 1-55648-141-1
      1. Medical statistics—Information services—United States—
Directories.   2. Hospitals—Information services—United States—
Directories.   3. Health planning—Handbooks, manuals, etc.   4. Health services administration—Handbooks, manuals, etc.   I. McKinnie, Diana B.
II. Young, Robert W.   III. Title.
RA407.3.F78   1995
362.1'1'0684—dc20   95-16417
                                                                        CIP

Catalog no. 127151

©1995 by American Hospital Publishing, Inc.,
an American Hospital Association company

Printed in the USA

ΛΗΛ is a service mark of the American Hospital Association used under license by American Hospital Publishing, Inc.

Text set in Palatino
3M—7/95—0415

Richard Hill, Senior Editor
Lee Benaka, Editor
Dennis Spaag, Editorial Assistant
Marcia Bottoms, Executive Editor
Peggy DuMais, Production Coordinator
Luke Smith, Cover Designer
Brian Schenk, Books Division Director

Contents

List of Figures and Tables

About the Authors

John D. Fry is the director of clinical services contracting for the University of Utah Faculty Practice Organization, Salt Lake City. The Faculty Practice Organization represents the 500 physicians of the University of Utah in their negotiations with managed care payers. In addition to managed care negotiations, Mr. Fry has developed joint ventures with payers for a new commercial HMO, a Medicaid HMO, and primary care clinics. In 1994, Mr. Fry worked with American Hospital Publishing to edit a book on capitation management targeted to hospital leadership. Prior to joining the University of Utah, Mr. Fry was a partner in Phase II Consulting, a health care management consulting firm.

Diana B. McKinnie is a graduate student in the medical informatics program at the School of Medicine at the University of Utah, Salt Lake City. Before returning to school, Ms. McKinnie was vice-president of a large medical software firm, where she was responsible for software development and customer support. She has published writings in the area of computerizing physician practices and has served as a consultant specializing in computers and outpatient practice for a firm based in Texas. Ms. McKinnie holds a bachelor of science degree from the University of California, Los Angeles, and a master of science degree from the University of Washington, Seattle.

Robert W. Young is president of the R. W. Young Management Group, a health care management consulting firm based in Salt Lake City. For more than 20 years, Mr. Young has provided clients throughout the United States, Canada, and Europe with strategic planning, market positioning, and financial feasibility services. In addition, he is extensively involved in developing integrated health care systems. Mr. Young holds a bachelor of science degree in accounting and a master's degree in business administration from the University of Utah, and he is a certified public accountant.

Prior to establishing an independent consulting practice, Mr. Young served as the national financial director of development for HCA Management Company, where he focused on the acquisition and operation of hospitals and management contract relationships throughout the United States. Mr. Young also served as vice-president for fiscal and data services for the Utah Hospital Association during the early 1980s.

Preface

In the authors' consulting engagements, it has been routine to go through a trial-and-error process of seeking hospital data from a particular state. It was during a particularly trying search that the idea for this book took form.

In 1992, American Hospital Publishing published the first edition of *The Health Care Data Source Book.* At the time, we anticipated that a second edition would be needed around 1997. Fortunately, the first edition was well received by health care professionals, and work started on this second edition in late 1993.

To say that the health care field is evolving rapidly is an understatement. The central theme of both editions of *The Health Care Data Source Book* is that the way a health care organization organizes, collects, and disseminates strategic market and planning data can either be a substantial asset or a substantial disadvantage. This edition of the book places the principles set forth in the first edition in the context of the current health care environment. To that end, information on payers is included, and the strategy control system is modified to accommodate vertically integrated delivery systems as well as fully integrated financing and delivery systems.

Fundamentally, this book is a resource to be used in the course of strategic planning and development of new services. The authors invite readers to alert them to additional sources of data that would be "naturals" to include in future editions. Please contact John Fry at the following address:

John D. Fry, Director, Clinical Services Contracting
School of Medicine, The University of Utah
127 South 500 East #110, Salt Lake City, UT 84102
(801) 297-4956 phone
(801) 297-4949 fax
e-mail: fry@edu-utah-med-fin

Acknowledgments

Many people deserve thanks for their direct and indirect participation in this book, not the least of whom are:

- "The Good Guys" (Tess Artig, R.N., Paulette Utz, Allison Kapp, Dan Lundergan, Neil Kochenour, M.D., Rick Fullmer, Gene Corapi, Cliff Hardesty, Christine St. Andre, and many others) at the University of Utah who create a "stimulating milieu" of discussion, unanswerable questions, and the occasional Zen-like health care financing riddle.
- The current and former Faculty Practice Organization board, including David Bragg, M.D., Marian Bishop, Ph.D., Harold Dunn, M.D., Bernie Grosser, M.D., Ric Harnsberger, M.D., John Holbrook, M.D., Rich Molteni, M.D., Chuck Norlin, M.D., Bill Odell, M.D., Ph.D., and James Parkin, M.D., for their unwavering commitment to "push the envelope."
- Lynn Simons, Ph.D., for his unwavering commitment to clear thought, clean living, and orderly approaches to blindingly complex projects.
- The members of the HEALTHMGMT electronic bulletin board developed, operated, and occasionally refereed by Jim Goes, Ph.D., of the University of Alaska Southeast, Juneau.

John also wishes to thank his coauthors, Diana McKinnie and Robert Young, without whom the second edition definitely would not have happened. Finally, John wishes to thank Vicki for "coverage" and Andy and Kit (ages 5 and 7) for letting him use "their computer." Also deserving of special thanks are John's parents D.L. and Dorothy Fry for their decades of support and encouragement.

Chapter 1

Introduction

As the health care field evolves, a key skill for any health care organization will be its ability to effectively use information, referred to herein as its information competence. This point may seem obvious; however, the notion of what constitutes *information skills* is evolving as the health care field evolves. In the past, useful information was often thought of as piles of computer paper, bound neatly and organized so that data generated by any department of the hospital could be readily located. A manager faced with making a decision needed only to access the reports in order to retrieve the facts desired. The availability of a wealth of computer-generated data may sound ideal, but it is only a part, and perhaps the least important part, of a health care organization's ability to effectively handle information.

High-level information skills encompass far more than the ability to use computers and telecommunications to gather ever-larger bases of data to be analyzed with increasing sophistication and presented with ever-more-dazzling graphics. In fact, an obsession with the amazing capabilities of computer hardware and software actually complicates achieving information competence. The mounds of data that can be created by even the simplest computer system complicate achieving information competence by:

- Focusing management attention on that which can be quantified (hard data can offer little or no support for many of the most important tasks of management; for example, a summarized attitude survey may identify physician morale problems but have little utility in solving them)
- Reinforcing the belief that huge amounts of data virtually guarantee solid decision making

A health care organization whose employees have highly developed information skills routinely has the necessary information to both control the organization's operations and anticipate and plan for major environmental shifts. Implicit in this statement is the assumption that the appropriate people in the organization have access to such information in a timely manner. Again, as obvious as that statement may seem, achieving the ideal in actuality is a tremendous undertaking.

The central theme of this book is that the *way* health care organizations manage information will either substantially help or substantially hinder them in the achievement of their goals. Furthermore, the management of information is much broader than the computerized generation of data. To this end, this book presents an example of a strategy control system and identifies multiple sources of strategic planning information.

Chapter 2 discusses information competence as a key to the successful operation of a health care organization. The most fundamental aspects of the health care field are undergoing unprecedented change. The way health care organizations use information will determine their future success.

Data overload is also discussed in chapter 2. It is safe to say that virtually every hospital administrator is experiencing data overload. The amazing capabilities of computer systems, coupled with the dizzying array of data available, make fertile ground for the provision of too much of the wrong type of data.

A solution to the data-overload problem begins to emerge through a concept known as the value of information. Applying value-of-information principles can help administrators focus on the specific information upon which an issue will turn.

To put the ideas discussed in chapter 2 into context, chapter 3 presents a methodology called the strategy control system. This methodology has been developed to routinely provide senior management with the information tools needed to manage the diverse goals of a typical health care organization.

The last chapter explains various recent techniques for data analysis. Among these techniques are the analysis of Medicare cost reports and utilization rate variances and the estimation of market size, market share, and health plan enrollments.

This book contains six appendixes. Appendixes A through C show which states make available particular inpatient, outpatient, and financial data that typically are of interest to hospital managers. Appendix D offers a directory of the principal sources within each state from which data indicated in the first three appendixes can be requested. A new appendix, appendix E, describes the basics of Internet access and lists electronic data resources (such as CD-ROMs, bulletin boards, databases, on-line journals, and user groups) and how to gain access to them. Appendix F provides an extensive list (by subject) of studies and reports of special interest to health care managers, as well as a list of the sources from which these studies and reports may be ordered.

Chapter 2

Information Skills as a Core Competency

A characteristic shared by virtually all successful companies in any type of business is the skilled use of information. In health care organizations, the skilled use of information is particularly important given the fundamental changes occurring in the health care field.

Factors Driving the Need for Information Competence

Some of the factors that drive the need for information competence in health care include the velocity of change and the impact of market-based changes.

The Velocity of Change

Change in the health care field is occurring on many fronts. However, technological advances and the increasing power of payers are two types of change that particularly complicate the management of hospitals and other health care organizations.

Technological advances in diagnosis and treatment have a substantial impact on how patient conditions are cared for. For example, it appears that in a few years there may be a vaccine that will prevent the Rous sarcoma virus (RSV) in children. Many children's hospitals and pediatric units see a marked increase in utilization in the winter and spring due to RSV. A vaccine will help eliminate such admissions. In addition, as of this writing phenomenal discoveries are occurring related to the genetic bases for diseases such as cystic fibrosis (CF). A genetic treatment will permanently affect the type of resources required to care for CF patients.

On the financial front, payers are becoming increasingly aggressive in their ability to influence provider choice. This is particularly apparent in the ability of large managed care payers to shift contracts from one group of providers to another. The speed at which this can affect hospital utilization is virtually unprecedented. Historically, only a natural disaster, a strike, or a fire could affect a hospital as dramatically as an aggressive payer. Being able to respond in a timely manner to the opportunities and threats that managed care presents is a good example of the use of high-level information skills.

The Impact of Market-Based Changes

The potential impact of legislatively driven health care reform rightly preoccupied those in health care financing and delivery during the early 1990s. Millions of hours of effort, many dollars, and countless sleepless nights were expended in positioning health care organizations for the anticipated effects of various health care reform proposals. As of this writing, it appears that only moderate legislative change will occur in the near future. Of much more interest and impact are the market-based changes which were, in large part, stimulated by concerns of legislative reform.

Market-based changes are proceeding at an astounding rate. For example, consider the following:

- Giant hospital systems are being created through mergers and acquisitions. The most notable example of the hospital system phenomenon is Columbia/HCA/Health Trust. In 1988 the Columbia system consisted of four hospitals. A scant seven years later, it is a behemoth with $11 billion in revenue, 197 hospitals and facilities, and a seemingly boundless commitment to the creation of integrated delivery systems.
- In nearly all metropolitan areas, physician organizations are forming in order to organize unaffiliated physicians into business entities. Perhaps the best example of physician organization is the Mullikin Group. The Mullikin Group is made up of 53 medical facilities in California, 400 physicians and other providers, and 3,000 support employees. In 1982, the Mullikin Group served 15,000 members; in 1994, it served over 300,000 members.
- Many hospitals and physician groups are pursuing integration so that they can offer a coordinated set of medical care delivery resources. Integration is being pursued through acquisitions (for example, hospitals buying physicians' practices) and through legal relationships where neither party owns the other (for example, physician–hospital organizations [PHOs]).
- The merger of hospital and physician services creates an integrated medical services delivery system. A more involved form of vertical

integration incorporates the medical care financing activity by linking a financing entity (insurer, HMO) with an integrated delivery entity. Perhaps the best known example of the fully integrated financing and delivery system is Kaiser Permanente.

A common thread running through virtually all of the market-based reform is an expansion in the scope of services that entities are responsible for delivering. Physician practices are expanding horizontally to provide convenient access to a larger population and vertically into outpatient centers to be able to accept responsibility for a wider range of services. Hospitals are expanding into ever bigger chains to gain economies of scale and to provide geographically convenient access. Hospitals are vertically integrating to provide physician services and health care financing services. Health care financing entities are gaining delivery capability.

Time will tell whether the various integration strategies described in the preceding list will ultimately be successful. However, to be sure, pursuing an integration strategy dramatically increases the scope of data the organization needs to guide its efforts and increases the sophistication with which the data must be interpreted. (Chapter 3 discusses the range of performance an organization must collect and measure and presents the idea of the strategy control system.)

The Development of Core Competencies

During the 1980s, the notion of *core competencies* began to appear in general management literature. Proponents argued that the general business environment changes too quickly for entities to be able to focus on attaining any reasonable degree of skill in providing a specific product or service. Instead, organizations would be better served by developing general skills (core competencies) that could be applied to future products and services as well as existing products and services.[1]

The way in which health care organizations use information may be considered a core competency. Information skills are a universal component of both routine and unusual hospital management issues. For all of the reasons mentioned earlier in this discussion, the effective acquisition, analysis, dissemination, and use of information is central to maximizing a health care organization's potential.

Several health care companies have excelled in a particular use of information. For example, American Hospital Supply (now Baxter Healthcare) created an automated ordering system known as ASAP in the early 1980s. This system was based on a personal computer and allowed users to order directly from American Hospital Supply. Today, the ASAP service is widely recognized as a strategic masterstroke that has helped this company maintain its position as a market leader.

Currently, effectiveness and efficiency measurements of hospitals are a cresting "environmental wave" that will crash on the health care field. Just as some commercial firms have developed methodologies for the hospital setting, so too have some firms developed similar measurement systems for physicians. Of course, the intended use of these types of systems is to identify effective and efficient providers and to direct patients to use them rather than other providers. Even if one ignores questions on the accuracy and validity of these measurement systems, it is clear that they are being used and will continue to be used as a basis for shifting patient flow from one group of providers to another. Woe be to the health care organization that is not actively attempting to manage quality (by whatever definition) and that does not have the information competencies to contest an unfavorable rating by commercial systems. A detailed discussion of the limitations of publicly available data in assessing hospital efficiency and effectiveness is contained in chapter 4.

The Control of Data Overload

One key aspect of effective and efficient use of data is that of gathering, analyzing, and disseminating information that will directly aid decision makers. In this process, it is easy to provide too much information, a condition commonly referred to as data overload. Health care is especially prone to data overload because of both its inherent complexity and the proliferation of computers in the health care field.

Health care delivery, especially the delivery of acute care services, is inherently complex. Consider the data needs and data generation of the various hospital entities and physicians involved in a routine outpatient surgery. With respect to hospital services, at least five departments (admitting, surgery, billing, laboratory, and radiology) are directly involved, and a host of others (for example, central supply) are peripherally involved. In addition to these hospital services, at least four physician specialties (surgery, anesthesiology, radiology, and pathology) are directly involved. Each of these nine entities needs some component of the total set of information generated to care for this patient. In addition, each of the nine entities contributes to the overall set of data associated with the patient.

The computerization of health care also contributes to the propensity for data overload. The computerization of hospitals has generally occurred on a department-by-department basis, a function-by-function basis, or both. This contributes to data overload in that each departmental or functional computer system generates its own set of reports. Typically, the individual reports are not combined as they move up the organizational hierarchy. The result is that senior management may receive numerous ancillary services reports when only a small percentage of the data in each report is needed. In addition, with the aid of computers, it is possible to generate a huge amount of data as well as analyses that would have been, for all practical purposes, impossible to generate manually.

When these factors are viewed together, it is easy to understand why health care is prone to data overload. A technique to determine the value of information, such as that covered in the next section, will help managers avoid data overload.

Ways to Determine the Value of Information

In a perfect world, all the facts pertinent to management decisions are readily available. Obviously, this ideal situation does not exist now and likely never will. One way to attempt to cope with a lack of information about a particular issue is to engage in heroic efforts to gather the information that is missing. In some circumstances, such heroic efforts can be justified by the potential magnitude of the issue at hand. However, usually it is impractical to attempt to eliminate the uncertainty that arises from a lack of complete information.

One reason the elimination of uncertainty is impractical is that the attainment of certainty requires a commitment of time. Some management scholars believe that the time an organization takes to accomplish goals is a key strategic variable. That is, the most successful firms in any industry will be able to develop products and services—and make changes in existing products and services—faster than their counterparts.[2] Obviously, the decision-making process an organization employs is a key determinant of the amount of time required to achieve goals.

Typically, a balance must be struck between committing time and resources to gather additional information and the incremental benefit afforded by the information being sought. An analytical concept known as the *value of information* can be used to help focus information-gathering efforts.

The following five guidelines will help health care managers determine the value of information being pursued and hence how much effort should be invested in gathering that information. The guidelines help managers prioritize the information that could be gathered, enabling them to devote resources to gathering information that will have the greatest impact on reaching a decision.

Focusing on Key Factors

First, managers should focus most of their efforts on gathering reliable information on the key factors that affect the decision.

One of the most important aspects of the value of information is the idea that not all information has equal value. In any circumstance requiring a decision, certain aspects of the circumstance have more impact on the resolution of the situation than others. Therefore, the key to determining where to expend resources is to identify the central issue or issues.

Focusing on the Level of the Decision

The second guideline is that the higher the level of decision, the greater the effort to minimize uncertainty.

Generally, business decisions can be positioned at three levels: the strategy level, the business unit level, and the department level. Strategy-level decisions are those that directly affect the entire organization. Examples of strategy-level decisions for a health care system include the following:

- Entering fundamentally new industries; for example, entering the health care financing field by creating a preferred provider organization (PPO) or a health maintenance organization (HMO)
- Expanding existing business unit services into a new geographic market; for example, acquiring a hospital in a neighboring city
- Creating a new business unit; for example, forming a company to develop and operate ambulatory surgery centers

Examples of business-unit–level decisions for a health care institution include the following:

- Adding additional bed capacity to an existing hospital
- Determining the size of the hospital's capital budget
- Increasing or decreasing the size of the hospital's staff

Examples of department-level decisions include the following:

- Allocating capital budget for a department among competing capital purchases
- Changing the vendors who supply the department with goods and services

Generally, the higher the decision level of a particular issue, the more information is required. Two factors drive this generality. First, high-level decisions generally affect the entire organization. Therefore, the risk of an error in decision making will have a broad-based impact. Second, higher-level decisions usually involve committing the organization to debt, consuming the organization's equity, or both. Therefore, the high-level decisions have financial consequences over relatively long time frames. As an example, consider the decision to add a new bed tower to a hospital. Once the bed tower is built, the hospital has irrevocably committed its resources. If that decision were in error, the practical recourse would be to try to convert the bed tower to some other productive use. In addition, the financial drain of a nonproductive bed tower would undoubtedly affect the ability of other parts of the hospital to secure resources.

Conversely, department-level decisions are made within set parameters (for example, the capital budget) and can generally be undone if a decision is found to be in error. For example, a decision to use a particular vendor can be changed quickly; or a piece of equipment can be resold if its performance is unsatisfactory. Although these decisions may be traumatic to the department manager, they will probably have little impact on the overall organization.

Focusing on the Number of Departments Affected

The third guideline is that the greater the number of departments operationally affected by a decision, the greater the need for certainty.

Because of the complexity of health care, as more hospital departments are affected by a potential decision, more information is needed to reduce the chance of inadvertently causing related problems in other departments should the decision be wrong. For example, assume the admissions office is determining which admissions software package to purchase. Because admissions information is used by many other departments in the hospital, it would be a potentially significant error not to have a high level of confidence in the adequacy of the software package being purchased. In effect, a mistake by the admissions office could have a direct impact on other departments in the hospital.

Focusing on the Difficulty of Reversing a Decision

The fourth guideline is that the more difficult it is to reverse a decision, the higher the level of confidence must be before making the decision.

When viewed objectively, many of the decisions made in a hospital management environment can be undone if the desired outcomes fail to materialize. Thus, these types of decisions can be made with relatively less certainty than those that cannot be undone.

However, a major barrier to acting on these types of situations is the management philosophy of the hospital's leadership. If the hospital administration has a reputation for punishing wrong judgments, it is highly likely that those in the position to make judgments will postpone them until every opportunity to minimize uncertainty has been taken.

Focusing on the Degree of Risk

The fifth guideline is that resources should be committed to obtaining information for decisions having the greatest risk.

One of the factors integral to the value of information is the cost of gathering information. It is easy to think that asking internal sources for information involves little cost because those personnel have to be paid regardless of whether they work on the information requested or on something else. However, there is an opportunity cost in using internal sources to gather additional data. Specifically, those personnel may be prevented from using that time to gather additional data on another activity that may be more valuable to the organization.

For example, assume that a financial analyst uses time to gather data that confirm the advisability of purchasing housekeeping equipment costing $5,000. Because the financial analyst was occupied with that project, an opportunity to save 1 percent of the annual cost of IV solutions was foregone. Obviously, the value to the organization of confirming the advisability of purchasing the equipment was far less than saving a fraction of the cost of IV solutions.

A System for Controlling the Flow of Information

To illustrate how the need for a wide variety of information can be met and yet tempered to avoid information overload, chapter 3 discusses three principles for the strategic control of information. It also offers guidelines for developing a useful information system and provides an example of a strategy control system in operation.

References

1. Prahalad, C. K., and Hamel, G. The core competence of the corporation. *Harvard Business Review* 3:79–93, May–June 1990.

2. Nevens, T. M., and others. Commercializing technology: what the best companies do. *Harvard Business Review* 3:154–63, May–June 1990.

Chapter 3

The Strategy Control System

The central idea behind the strategy control system is that information routinely provided to management should correspond with the strategic objectives and goals of the organization. Such management-directed information, which is subsequently used to control the organization, has a substantial impact on organizational behavior. There is more than a grain of truth in the saying, "What you measure is what you get." An organization that unwittingly emphasizes the achievement of financial goals will almost certainly find that other important goals go wanting.

Currently, most organizations provide their managers with highly detailed financial information, but information about other objectives and goals may be provided only sporadically or not at all. Business organizations have tended to focus information-gathering efforts on financial measures and accounting systems. This is primarily a function of the needs of the financial community. For example, debt holders require financial information on the security of their holdings, and firms having publicly traded stock must comply with Securities and Exchange Commission regulations concerning the disclosure of financial status. Although financial information is obviously very important, it is by no means the only source of information that management requires. Furthermore, financial information can be seductive in its apparent objectivity and completeness.[1]

The idea of a strategy control system or a balanced scorecard fits health care organizations very well. Hospitals and other providers are by their very nature extremely complex economic entities. Integrated delivery organizations are even more complex; integrated delivery and financing systems approach being "off the scale" in terms of their economic complexity. Inherent economic complexity is exacerbated by reorganizations, mergers and acquisitions, technological change in the care process, and so forth. The following section on gathering information for a balanced scorecard in a business environment takes a look at some strategic issues that confront health care organizations as they develop a strategy control system.

A Balanced Scorecard Approach

In their article "Putting the Balanced Scorecard to Work," Robert S. Kaplan and David P. Norton discuss how three firms, Rockwater (a division of Brown & Root/Haliburton that provides underwater construction services), Apple Computer, and Advanced Micro Devices, developed and use the balanced scorecard. The process to develop the balanced scorecard described by Kaplan and Norton is similar to the steps that follow in this chapter to develop a strategy control system. To wit: start with the vision of the organization as translated into its strategy and identify specific measurements that correspond to four areas:

- *Financial measurements* are largely the traditional measures of profitability, returns, and so forth.
- *Customer measurements* focus on how well the firm knows its markets and customers.
- *Internal measurements* include effectiveness, efficiency, quality, and so forth.
- *Growth measurements* focus on progress in service innovation, the proportion of revenue coming from new services, and like measures.

In addition to the relatively straightforward measurements discussed above, customized indexes of competitive pricing, rate of improvement, customer satisfaction, and so forth can be developed.

Kaplan and Norton sum up the idea of the balanced scorecard and the strategy control system:

> The balanced scorecard is not a template that can be applied to businesses in general or even industry-wide. Different market situations, product strategies, and competitive environments require different scorecards. . . . In fact, a critical test of a scorecard's success is its transparency: from the 15 to 20 scorecard measures, an observer should be able to see through to the business unit's competitive strategy.[2]

A basic premise of management is that an organization's strategy must match its opportunities in the market, which are in large part a function of its financial and nonfinancial assets, its capabilities. Once an organization's strategy has been set, it can go about organizing its resources to create the product or service envisioned in its strategy. In all but the smallest of organizations competing in stable industries, monitoring and controlling the enterprise must be done through a systematized flow of information. By managing the flow of information, the organization can adjust its operations to more nearly match the demands of the market.

Although the necessity for this flow of data may sound obvious, in a fast-moving field such as health care collecting and using the right set of information is much trickier than it sounds. Peter Drucker, writing in a *Wall Street Journal* editorial entitled "Be Data Literate—Know What to Know," put it this way:

> But the organization also has to become information literate. It also needs to learn to ask: What information do we need in this company? When do we need it? In what form? And where do we get it? So far, such questions are being asked primarily by the military, and even there mainly for tactical, day-to-day decisions. In business such questions have been asked only by a few multinationals, foremost among them the Anglo-Dutch Unilever, a few oil companies such as Shell, and the large Japanese trading companies.
>
> The moment these questions are asked, it becomes clear that the information a business most depends on is available, if at all, only in primitive and disorganized form. For what a business needs the most for its decisions—especially its strategic ones—are data about what goes on outside of it. It is only outside the business where there are results, opportunities and threats.[3]

Information literacy for managers in the health care field is becoming an ever-more-challenging proposition because of the extensive change the delivery and financing of health care is undergoing. The strategy control system provides a ready framework for management to create an information literacy framework.

Three Principles of Strategy Control

Generally, health care organizations have broad-ranging strategic objectives and goals—from meeting the health care needs of their community, to ensuring their financial viability, to providing the highest-quality patient care. Obviously, in order to manage the various goals and objectives of the health care organization, managers must routinely have information about the status of each. The strategy control system is based on three principles: appropriate information, organized information, and timely information.

Principle One: Appropriate Information

As stated at the beginning of this chapter, information routinely provided to management should correspond with the overall strategic goals and objectives of the organization.

Most hospitals include the delivery of high-quality care as a cornerstone in their strategic plan or their mission statement. Under a strategy control system, information on the quality of care would routinely be presented to management at all levels. Further, the information would not be simply of an "exception" nature, such as that of incident reports and so forth.

Principle Two: Organized Information

Information generated by the strategy control system should flow through a health care organization in an organized manner.

Generally, hospitals have highly organized methods for gathering and disseminating financial and, to a lesser extent, utilization information. However, other types of information usually are gathered in a less structured manner. A central tenet of the strategy control system is that most areas of the hospital should contribute both financial and nonfinancial data and information to the hospital system.

A particular department of the hospital (for example, the planning and marketing department) is responsible for aggregating, analyzing, and preparing summary reports. Nearly all parts of the hospital will, in turn, receive information from the strategy control system. The format of the reports from the system should be standardized. This standardization allows users of the reports to quickly assimilate information.

Principle Three: Timely Information

The strategy control system should receive, generate, and disseminate information on an established timetable.

It is not unusual to have some types of important management information developed on an ad hoc basis. The departments contributing data and information to the system will know precisely what information is expected and when it is due. In turn, the various parts of the health care organization will also know when reports are due back to them.

Developing a Strategy Control System

The end result of the strategy control system is to routinely provide all levels of hospital management with both the specific and general background information needed to resolve routine management issues. In addition, the system allows management to anticipate and respond to major environmental changes. The next part of this chapter puts the three principles into context for a typical hospital.

Identifying the Data and Information to Be Collected

The first step in developing a strategy control system is to review the hospital's strategic plan in order to identify objectives and goals. As mentioned earlier in this chapter, management routinely needs to have information that will enable it to manage *all* of the hospital's objectives and goals, not just its financial ones. This information can generally be grouped into three categories:

- *Information generated within the hospital:* Such internal data include the following: financial performance indicators, volume/utilization measures, key cost factors, key productivity factors, measures of quality, and measures of physician, employee, and patient satisfaction.
- *Context information on the local market:* Local market information includes: market size and market share of entities competing with the hospital, the size of health plans in terms of member/employee enrollment, and a summary of the status of legislative efforts that would affect the hospital.
- *General strategic planning information:* Such planning information includes: hospital utilization on a national basis, the status of proposed changes in Medicare and Medicaid legislation, and the status of other health care legislation, such as state-level or national health plan efforts. In addition, strategic planning information includes technological changes that will create a change in the way specific services are delivered. Changes in payer policies regarding the way in which services are reimbursed are also included in this area.

To illustrate the link between a hospital's objectives, goals, and needs for information, the example in figure 3-1 has been structured in the context of a major tertiary care hospital in a community where other hospitals are actively seeking potential patients. In addition, the example has been designed around the particular needs of senior management. The figure lists six institutional goals and objectives, as well as the institution's choices for information to be collected and managed.

Most of the internal information a hospital needs is generated at the department level. For example, financial and volume/utilization information can be most easily accessed from whatever computer system(s) serve the department. Similarly, key cost factors, key productivity factors, and measures of quality can all be based on data generated within the department.

Measures of community, physician, and patient satisfaction are best done on a hospitalwide basis. High-quality survey design and administration is a deceptively difficult task that requires specialized expertise.

Figure 3-1. Sample Information Collection Targets for Chosen Goals and Objectives of a Major Tertiary Care Hospital

Objective:	To serve our extended community by providing the highest-quality patient care regardless of a patient's ability to pay
Information to Manage:	• Measurement of community satisfaction with hospital services
	• Measurement of quality of patient care, including mortality rates, readmissions, nosocomial infections, and possible use of commercial-quality assessment services
	• Target rates of charity care in terms of patient volume, as well as gross charges for services
Objective:	To anticipate and implement plans to accommodate changes in health care delivery and financing
Information to Manage:	• Status of national, state, and local health care legislative efforts
	• National trends in hospital utilization
	• Status of proposed changes in Medicare and Medicaid legislation
	• Update on technological advances that will affect the manner in which diagnosis and therapy occur
	• Effect on hospital's finances if "best practice" techniques were currently done on most common diagnosis-related groups
Objective:	To ensure the financial viability of the hospital by achieving the average surplus attained by similar hospitals
Information to Manage:	• Overall hospital income statement and department-level income statements
	• Analysis of volume by total hospital and by department
	• Analysis of key productivity factors by department
	• Analysis of key cost factors by department
	• Analysis of effective reimbursement by top managed care contractors compared to full average cost of service delivery
Objective:	To continue our position as the leading tertiary care facility in our market area by increasing the proportion of patients we serve by the early adoption of proven clinical techniques
Information to Manage:	• Market share of admissions for the entire hospital and by department
Objective:	To serve a larger portion of patients from the most desirable managed care organizations
Information to Manage:	• Analysis of payers in terms of size and financial characteristics and share of patients served
Objective:	To be the hospital having the most complete clinical technology as measured by physicians' perceptions
Information to Manage:	• Physician survey

By having surveys performed on a hospitalwide basis, numerous pitfalls can be avoided, such as selecting an inappropriate survey method, creating a survey instrument that measures the wrong set of variables, or administering the survey in a manner that results in a skewed response.

Context information on the local market largely results from internal analyses. These include estimates of market size, market share, and the size of health plans, as well as analysis of legislative efforts. Chapter 4 briefly describes the issues associated with estimating market size, market share, and health plan enrollments.

General strategic planning information is readily available to the reader. A number of publications are listed in the appendixes of this book. They track general trends in hospital utilization, changes in reimbursement, and other health care legislative initiatives such as any efforts to establish a national health plan. Examples of specific sources of information are listed in table 3-1.

Identifying the Means of Collecting the Information

The next step in the development of a strategy control system is to identify the means of collecting the information required by the hospital to fulfill its goals and objectives. In terms of collecting data on the local market and general strategic planning, the references and external sources in the appendixes should prove extremely useful.

Tapping the sources of data generated internally should also be a relatively straightforward task. However, managers may encounter difficulties in generating data in the ideal format if the hospital's computer systems are relatively inflexible in their report-generation capability.

Two practical aspects of internal data collection require significant attention. First, managers must determine exactly how each performance variable should be measured. Even such apparently simple measures as the number of outpatient visits for a particular department need definition. For example, does the number of outpatient visits counted include only those visits that are billed? If this definition is used, follow-up surgical visits for which there is no charge should not be included in the count.

The second aspect of internal data collection that requires the manager's attention is the potential inconsistency in the way variables are measured from one time period to another. For example, department managers who have been involved in generating detailed volume and productivity data probably had to make judgment calls regarding the way particular variables are to be measured. Assuming that those decisions are sound, they should be institutionalized in a formal procedure so that consistent data measurement will continue should the current manager be assigned duties elsewhere.

Table 3-1. Sample Chart for Locating Information and Assigning Responsibility

Information Need	Data Source	Timetable	Position Responsible
Community satisfaction survey	Survey	Annually	Vice-president (VP) planning/marketing
Quality of patient care: • Mortality/ morbidity • Readmissions • Nosocomial infections	Internal data, Centers for Disease Control	Measured monthly, compared annually	Chief operating officer (COO)
Quality of patient care: • Patient satisfaction	Patient satisfaction	Semiannually	VP planning/marketing
Charity care	Income statement, volume analysis	Monthly	COO
Financial viability	Hospital and department income statement	Monthly	Chief financial officer (CFO)
Financial viability	Hospital and department key cost factor analysis	Monthly	CFO
Financial viability	Hospital and department volume analysis	Monthly	COO
Financial viability	Hospital and department productivity factor analysis	Monthly	COO
Effect of "best" practice	Practice protocols	Annually (COO/CFO)	COO/CFO
Managed care reimbursement	Reimbursement and cost-accounting data	Semiannually	CFO
Market position	Market share of admits	Quarterly	VP planning/marketing
Managed care share	Analysis of payers	Semiannually	CFO
Managed care share	Share of patients	Semiannually	VP planning/marketing
Clinical technology	Survey of physicians	Annually	VP planning/marketing
Legislative efforts	Hospital associations, trade publications, newsletters	As needed, but at least annual update	VP planning/marketing
National hospital utilization	American Hospital Association (AHA)	Annually	VP planning/marketing
Medicare/Medicaid	Hospital associations, trade publications, newsletters	As needed, but at least annual update	VP planning/marketing
Technological advances	AHA, trade publications	Quarterly	VP planning/marketing

Identifying the Timetable and Assigning Responsibility

Because hospitals are such complex business entities, a data system will easily founder if a realistic timetable for the collection and dissemination of information is not established and adhered to. An overlooked aspect of the quality of information is its timeliness. Receiving information too late to affect a decision is, in some ways, worse than not receiving the information at all.

An additional but important aspect of data dissemination is that different levels of the organization will receive information with different levels of detail. For example, the manager of respiratory therapy needs to have a line-item accounting of all expenses, whereas senior management needs only general summary information about respiratory therapy. Information dissemination should ensure that each manager receives information that is pertinent but not overloaded with detail appropriate to a lower level of the organization.

In terms of making the data system work, perhaps no other aspect is as important as clearly assigning the authority and responsibility for data collection, as well as the timetable upon which the data system will function. The chart in table 3-1 summarizes the information item to be reviewed, the timing for completing reports to be passed up through the organizational structure, the source of the data, and the position responsible for the analysis and production of each report.

Internal Distribution by Electronic Systems

As mentioned earlier, timely collection and distribution of strategy control data is extremely important. Data not available in time to influence a management decision are essentially useless. In addition, the whole idea behind the strategy control system is to create a real-time source of critical management information. If the system is not operationally fluid, it will be hard to gain the wholehearted commitment of the individuals supplying information and those using the information. One means to help achieve a fluid system is to base the collection and distribution of information around an electronic mail (e-mail) system.

One of the devilish challenges to senior management is how to keep constituencies, especially employees and physicians, informed about what is happening. There have been reams written on the value of keeping employees and physicians informed and educated about "what's going on." However, the practical problem of communicating by paper or in person is huge, particularly in a health care organization that cannot just "stop production" and call everyone to an auditorium. Electronic mail can be an extremely useful means to routinize communication of the strategy control system. The routine, real-time updates possible with e-mail will help intertwine the strategy control system (and hence the organization's mission, strategy, and goals) with line employees and the management team.

How the Evolving Health Care System Affects the Strategy Control System

The fundamental premise of the strategy control system is to routinely provide the range of data necessary to monitor the organization's strategy and objectives. Currently, the health care field is in the midst of fundamental reorganization. Many hospitals are increasing the scope of their services to include outpatient facilities and professional services. Some physician groups are buying or building their own facilities. Hospitals and physicians are creating health care financing services such as HMOs and PPOs. Payers are buying and building health care delivery resources. Given the rate of environmental change, keeping the strategy control process consistent with the organization's strategy and objectives requires diligence.

Earlier in this chapter, an illustration of the strategy control system for a "traditional" tertiary care hospital was developed. To demonstrate how the strategy control system changes when a hospital's strategy changes, this section develops additional data needed for two "generic" hospital strategies. The two generic strategies are:

- *Integrated health care delivery system strategy:* This assumes vertical integration within the range of health care service delivery. Vertical service delivery integration includes inpatient and outpatient facility services, primary care, and multispecialty physician services. Figure 3-2 and table 3-2 describe the additional information requirements, data sources, timetables, and individual responsible for handling the information.
- *Integrated health care delivery and financing system strategy:* In addition to a full range of service delivery resources, this strategy adds financing capability in the form of owned HMOs, PPOs, insurance companies, and so forth.

If an organization pursues the fully integrated strategy of offering both a full range of services and financing capability, the strategy control information requirements become even more complex. Specifically, in addition to all the information listed earlier for the tertiary care and integrated delivery system, the fully integrated financing and delivery system needs HEDIS information, additional financial and revenue information, and standard value measures. (See figure 3-3 and table 3-3.) These two examples show that as a hospital's strategy expands, the type of information that will need to be routinely collected, analyzed, and distributed expands dramatically in scope.

Figure 3-2. Additional Information Needed to Support an Integrated Delivery System Strategy

Objective:	To operate our outpatient facilities and professional offices with a high level of efficiency and patient satisfaction
Information to Manage:	• Measurement of patient satisfaction at each component of integrated delivery system
	• Comparison of patient satisfaction at owned outpatient facilities and professional offices versus patient satisfaction at private professional offices
Objective:	To retain at least 90% of referrals from owned professional offices within the integrated system
Information to Manage:	• Analysis of number and type of referrals staying within integrated system
Objective:	To have either owned or contracted primary care professional offices geographically convenient to 50% of the population of our market area
Information to Manage:	• Comparison of population data to office locations
Objective:	To ensure the financial viability of the system by maintaining at least the average return on assets achieved by similar systems
Information to Manage:	• Standard financial ratio analysis with particular attention on return-on-asset measures
	• Analysis of utilization and cost of services at outpatient facilities and visits at professional offices

Table 3-2. Sample Chart for Additional Information for Integrated Delivery System

Information Need	Data Source	Timetable	Position Responsible
Patient satisfaction planning/marketing	Ongoing survey	Monthly	Vice-president (VP)
Comparison of satisfaction	Survey of other systems' patients	Annually	VP planning/marketing
Referrals in system	Operational data	Monthly	Chief operating officer (COO)
Convenience of offices	U.S. Census data	Annually	VP planning/marketing
Financial ratios	Operational data	Monthly	Chief financial officer
Cost/volume services	Operational data	Monthly	COO

Information Skills for Serving Community Needs

A graphic way to describe the importance of information skills is to imagine management issues as having velocity. Only a decade ago, issues surfaced and progressed toward the decision maker in a predictable fashion. They could be analyzed and plans for action drawn up in a relatively relaxed manner. The velocity and complexity of issues have increased dramatically. Changes in clinical technology are being developed

Figure 3-3. Sample Information Collection Targets for a Fully Integrated Delivery and Financing System

Objective:	To operate our health care financing services efficiently, effectively, and with a high level of member satisfaction
Information to Manage:	• HEDIS 2.0 measurement system
	• Measurement of effective financial yield of owned financial services to contracted HMOs and PPOs
	• Measurement of member satisfaction
Objective:	To obtain a growing share of system revenue from owned financial services
Information to Manage:	• Analysis of proportion of revenue from owned financial services compared to other managed care contracts
Objective:	To have superior value in our financial services
Information to Manage:	• A standard measurement of benefits, cost, and member satisfaction of owned financial services and other health plans

Table 3-3. Sample Chart for Additional Information for Fully Integrated Delivery and Financing System

Information Need	Data Source	Timetable	Position Responsible
HEDIS analysis	Operational data	Quarterly	Vice-president (VP) financing services
Financial yield	Analysis of reimbursement by managed care plans	Quarterly	Chief financial officer (CFO)
Member satisfaction	Survey	Semiannually	Vice-president (VP) planning/marketing
Proportion of revenue	Analysis of reimbursement by managed care plans	Annually	CFO
Standard value measure	Market survey data, member satisfaction survey	Annually	VP planning/marketing

and brought to market faster than ever before. Managed care payers can shift literally thousands of admissions from one group of providers to another in a matter of weeks.

One consequence of the complexity and increased velocity of issues is that the time frame in which an effective response must be developed is being reduced. The slack time to gather background information and analyze data is being eliminated. Having the information needed to respond to all but the most unusual of circumstances constitutes a new form of competency in truly serving the needs of the patient population.

References

1. Eccles, R. G. The performance measurement manifesto. *Harvard Business Review* 69(1):131–37, Jan.–Feb. 1991.

2. Kaplan, R. S., and Norton, D. P. Putting the balanced scorecard to work. *Harvard Business Review* 71(5):134–43, Sept.–Oct. 1993.

3. Drucker, P. F. Be data literate—know what to know. *Wall Street Journal*, Dec. 1, 1992, p. A16.

Chapter 4

Applications and Techniques for Information Analysis

Although the ways that any one health care organization can use internally and externally generated data are almost limitless, there are a few applications from which virtually all health care organizations can benefit. This chapter discusses several ways to analyze information and to put into practice many of the ideas discussed in the preceding chapters.

The first application is a Medicare cost report analysis. Medicare cost reports have the virtue of being the only common description of utilization and economic activity for hospitals in the United States. As such, they can be used as a least common denominator for comparing one facility to another.

The second application is the estimation of market size. The determination of market size is an essential element in making many types of high-level decisions. For example, before committing scarce capital and human resources to the development of a new clinical program, it only makes sense to measure the demand for the program being considered.

The third application is the analysis of utilization rate variance. Clearly, a dominant theme of the 1990s is the attempt to reduce the variation in the amount of health care consumed for a given condition. Utilization rate variance is key to determining whether the health care providers in a given area are relatively heavy or light users of a particular procedure.

The authors are indebted to Brent L. Rufener for writing this chapter's discussion on monitoring the political process. Mr. Rufener is director, provider relations, for O.D.S. Health Plan in Portland, Oregon. Before joining O.D.S. Health Plan, Mr. Rufener was a principal at Phase II Consulting in Salt Lake City, Utah. He has also served as the chief lobbyist for the Utah Medical Association, where he directed legislative relations at both the state and federal levels. He received his master's degree in economics from the University of North Carolina at Chapel Hill.

The fourth application, estimating market share for certain individual hospitals as well as for all hospitals serving a given area, is central to identifying segments of a community that may be underserved. Similarly, estimating managed care health plan enrollment, the fifth application, is crucial because enrollment levels can dramatically alter a given hospital's market share.

The final section of this chapter discusses practical guidelines for monitoring the political process, that is, for acquiring information that can shed light on changes in government reimbursement and other variables affecting the local market for health care services. No other arena of human endeavor has the capability to so significantly alter the environment in which hospitals exist, particularly in light of the myriad health care reforms now being debated in state and federal circles.

Analyzing Medicare Cost Reports

Medicare cost reports filed annually by hospitals are an often-overlooked source of valuable information about a hospital's operations and market position. Even though most hospitals are reimbursed by Medicare for inpatient services under the prospective payment system (that is, according to diagnosis-related groups, or DRGs), hospitals are required to file annual cost reports in much the same way as they did before the advent of DRGs. Cost reports are available to the public under the Freedom of Information Act and can be obtained through the local Medicare intermediary (for example, Blue Cross or Aetna). The specific sources of information for each state are included in the first four appendixes of this book. Because the process for obtaining a report requires a written request, notification of the provider, and other processing requirements, it may take several months to obtain a report.

In some respects, cost reports are similar to tax returns. Specifically, there are detailed guidelines for the compilation and disclosure of information, and the end purpose of the reports is to determine the financial obligation of the Health Care Financing Administration (HCFA) to the provider.

Like tax returns, cost reports can be subject to aggressive gamesmanship by both the hospital and HCFA. For example, a provider could attempt to maximize the allocation of costs to areas with disproportionately high Medicare utilization. Under today's payment system of DRGs for inpatients and cost-based reimbursement for outpatients, the hospital has the incentive to maximize the allocation of costs to areas of high Medicare outpatient utilization. These biases should be kept in mind when utilizing cost report data.

Examples of several useful types of data that can be extracted from a cost report include the following:

- Gross utilization (beds, discharges, patient days, and so forth)
- Utilization by major hospital units (general medical/surgical units, intensive care units, and so forth)
- Data on the utilization by Medicare/Medicaid patients versus patients not served by government payment programs
- Breakdown of each cost center's expenses (surgery, radiology, laboratory, or other cost centers) into salaries and other expenses
- Identification of charges by cost center, which in conjunction with expenses by cost center provides some insight into the provider's pricing markup strategies and direct-cost margin by department
- Identification of remunerations paid to hospital-based physicians by type of service (radiology, laboratory, anesthesiology, and so forth)
- Identification of existing and new capital costs (increased investment in building and equipment, for example)

Annual cost reports provide a fairly detailed view of the financial operations of the hospitals serving a particular market. Assimilation of the available data on an annual basis for all providers in a given market area can provide valuable insight into how a particular facility compares to others. In essence, cost report analysis provides one more piece in the puzzle to achieve a better understanding of the health care marketplace.

Estimating Market Size

Market size can be estimated in two ways. The easiest but potentially most misleading way is simply to access utilization information collected by a state agency regarding the historical volume for a particular market segment for each hospital in the market area and to aggregate the information to reach a total market size. However, this method generally has two significant drawbacks. First, it ignores patient in-migration and out-migration. Suppose, for example, that there is a need to measure the frequency of cardiovascular surgery in a market area with two 100-bed community hospitals and a population of 50,000. Given the small size of both facilities, on the surface it is safe to assume that a large portion of cardiovascular procedures is being referred out of the market area to facilities having greater clinical depth. Therefore, simply measuring the number of cardiovascular procedures performed at the two hospitals would greatly understate the size of the market.

The second drawback to this method of measuring market size is that it is inherently reactive. Most states have a significant lag time in collecting, compiling, and making data available to the public. It is not unusual that data collected two years earlier are the most recent available. Relying on two-year-old data may result in identifying changes in market size long after they have actually occurred and thus providing a delayed and probably ineffectual response to a legitimate community need.

A better way to measure market size is to apply utilization rates to current and projected estimates of population by age and sex cohorts. Establishing the base data for this method requires more initial effort but generally provides far superior results. Two types of data are needed to generate an estimate of market size using this method: population by age and sex cohorts and utilization rates by diagnosis code, age, and sex.

Unless a demographic consultant is retained, the best population data are generally available from state government agencies. Generally, the most reliable estimates of state and local populations are provided by the economic analysis bureaus of state governments. In addition, some universities have departments that periodically update estimates of population. The U.S. Census Bureau also provides generally reliable estimates; however, state and university sources are able to more quickly incorporate changes in factors that affect local populations. The most convenient sources of census data are the 1,400 federal depository libraries, which generally are found in university or college libraries.

For larger metropolitan areas, municipal government agencies may also have reliable population data. Population estimates are also available from private firms specializing in the generation of market research information. As a general rule, population data generated from entities having a vested interest in data that show high-growth expectations should be avoided. For example, local economic development entities, private and public, are notorious for making optimistic projections.

Utilization rates by diagnosis code, age, and sex require raw data analysis. As indicated in the appendixes of this book, several states collect detailed patient discharge records, including such data as patient diagnosis, age, and sex. Whenever possible, these data should be obtained in an electronic format so that the user can easily analyze the number of diagnoses of a particular condition by age and sex. The diagnosis count can then be annualized (most states only collect a time-specific sample of data) and then compared to the population count in a particular cohort in order to obtain an incidence rate. Incidence rates are generally expressed in terms of the number of cases per 1,000 or 10,000 population. The incidence rate is then applied to the population in a particular hospital's service area to determine total market size.

Analyzing Utilization Rate Variances

As mentioned in the preceding section, fortunate hospitals may have access to detailed diagnosis information in an electronic format for their own states. However, regardless of whether electronic data are available for a particular state, comparing the utilization rates of a number of states can be very revealing.

Comparing utilization rates across states can reveal startling differences in incidence and other factors such as length of stay. For example, it is generally thought that California hospitals are relatively efficient due, in part, to long exposure to sophisticated managed care payers. Thus, if the frequencies of controversial procedures such as back surgery or coronary artery bypass grafts exceed those in comparison states for a particular market, it would be reasonable to expect utilization of those services in California to fall over an extended period of time.

The following paragraphs contain actual comparisons for three types of procedures. These comparisons illustrate variations in utilization from state to state, city to city, and region to region.

Sample Utilization Rate Variances

Back-surgery procedures (DRGs 214 and 215) are among the most common surgical procedures performed in the United States. Yet the usage from one area to another varies widely. For example, the rates of surgery in the Salt Lake City, Utah, and Columbus, Ohio, markets are almost two-thirds higher than in the San Diego, California, market, as displayed in figure 4-1.

Even within a given state, the variances in usage of a common imaging procedure (for example, CT scanning) can vary substantially. For

Figure 4-1. Back-Surgery Utilization Rates (Variance by City)

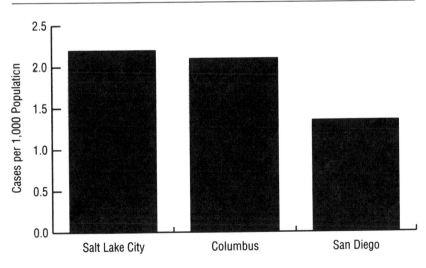

Source: R. W. Young Management Group.

example, in California 36 percent more CT examinations are given to people living in San Francisco than to those living in the San Jose market area less than 50 miles away (see figure 4-2).

On the other hand, variances in cholecystectomy (gallbladder removal, a common surgical procedure) from one region of the United States to another is relatively moderate. The extreme ends of the range in utilization rates vary by only 6 percent above and below the national average (see figure 4-3).

Causes of Variation in Utilization Rates

Variations in utilization and prevalence rates beg the obvious question: why? Many factors contribute to variations in data and rates:

- Differences in the demographic characteristics of the population served
- Differences in the community's standards of medical practice
- Differences in the practice style of area physicians
- Differences in the diagnostic and therapeutic resources available
- Degree of medical entrepreneurship and aggressive medical ventures in the market area
- Degree and volume of managed care in the market area

The differences in utilization rates attributable to different demographic characteristics of the population can be minimized by developing

Figure 4-2.   CT Scan Utilization Rates (Variance by California Cities)

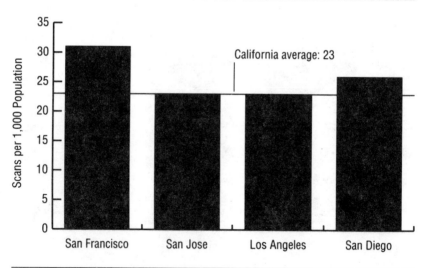

Source: R. W. Young Management Group.

Figure 4-3. Cholecystectomy Utilization Rates (Variance by Region of the United States)

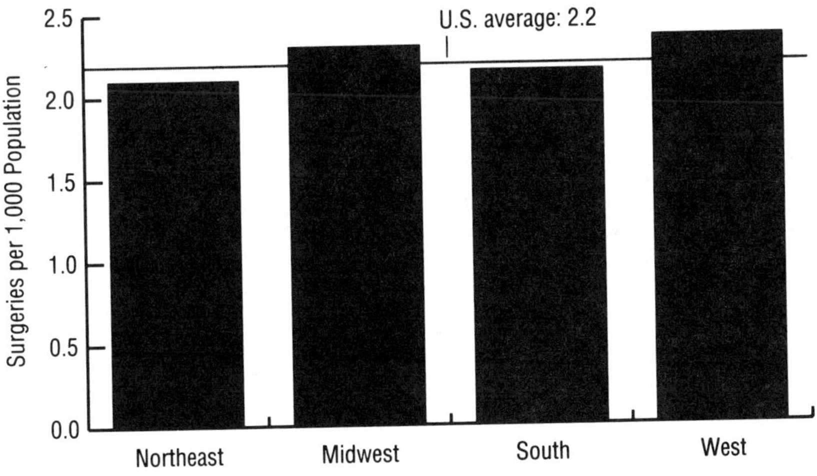

Source: R. W. Young Management Group.

age-specific use rates. Again, data in an electronic format are necessary, and obviously one of the data elements collected must be the age of the patient.

All these factors have varying degrees of impact on the actual utilization of medical services. Aside from variations in actual utilization, another major factor to be considered is the difference between a *facility use rate* and a *resident use rate*.

Facility Use Rate

When individuals living in a certain geographic area receive only a portion of their health care from providers in that area, this can substantially confound the development of a use rate. The most easily developed use rate is the facility use rate. A facility use rate is based on the utilization of a particular medical service or procedure at facilities within a given market area. The utilization is then divided by the population within the same area. For example, the number of open-heart procedures done in the state of Missouri divided by the population of Missouri results in the facility use rate for open-heart procedures for hospitals in Missouri.

The principal risk of blindly using these data is that they are subject to the impact of patient in-migration and out-migration in the area. In the context of the Missouri example, the facility use rate would not include residents of Kansas City, Missouri, who received open-heart surgery in hospitals in Kansas City, Kansas. Generally, large regional referral centers tend to have inflated utilization rates, and outlying rural facilities tend to have deflated rates. The more heterogeneous a market is compared to its surrounding markets, the greater the variation in use rate.

Resident Use Rate

A resident use rate is a more accurate reflection of the use of medical services by a population living in a given area. It is calculated by accumulating the usage of a given service from all providers, regardless of their location, that care for patients living in a given area. However, this information is generally available only from states with data commissions or state reporting requirements or from national surveys. Again, using the Missouri example, ideally the states surrounding Missouri would have the home addresses of open-heart surgery patients. On the basis of that information, the number of Missouri residents who have undergone surgery in Kansas (and other states) could be determined. Unfortunately, such ideal circumstances are rarely encountered.

Both facility and resident use rates can provide invaluable insights. It is critical, however, to understand the limits and uses of both. Ideally, access to both rates allows users the ability to assess the actual usage of services by the population served, as well as the relative market strengths and weaknesses of area providers in influencing patient in-migration and out-migration.

Estimating Market Share

Once the size of a particular market has been determined and the factors causing any significant variances in utilization (such as in-migration and out-migration) have been taken into account, the market share of various entities within a defined area can be estimated with relative ease. Again, fortunate hospitals have access to state-collected, diagnosis-specific data that can be used to measure any hospital's volume directly.

If such data are not available, estimates can be based on the only data point that is known for certain, specifically, the volume of the user's own hospital. Through an iterative process, the market share of other hospitals in the market area can be estimated by using this information. For example, if only the size of a market and a single hospital's volume are known, the market shares of other hospitals can be estimated based on the number of operating beds at each of the other hospitals. Admittedly, this is a gross measure at best; however, other data, such as the number of physicians in a particular specialty on staff at a particular hospital, can be used to further refine the estimate.

Obviously, estimating market shares without reliable data requires making a series of judgments, and judgments by definition are not always accurate. However, from a management perspective most of the value of maintaining estimates of market share over time is in the relative changes among area hospitals, not in the absolute estimates. For example, estimates showing a constant number of orthopedic cases over time would not be cause for alarm. However, estimates showing the market share of orthopedic cases falling in a growing market would generally be cause for some sort of management action. Therefore, a critical aspect of creating usable market share information is to use the same judgment system over time so that even when the market share estimates are flawed, they are flawed in a consistent manner.

Estimating Health Plan Enrollment

The size of various health plan enrollments is relatively easy to obtain by simply calling the various plans in a given market and asking for their current total enrollment. However, care must be taken to clarify the basis upon which enrollment is counted. Health maintenance organizations and preferred provider organizations (PPOs) generally base their enrollment counts on their *members,* which include all employees and dependents enrolled in the health plan. Employers with self-funded plans and insurers generally report only the number of employees enrolled in the plan.

In addition, most state insurance departments require that health insurers and HMOs file annual reports. Sometimes annual reports explicitly include the number of insured persons or members. If such figures are not available, an estimate can be calculated by dividing total premiums by an estimate of the average premium per insured person or member.

Measuring the Relative Effectiveness and Efficiency of Hospitals

A number of commercial organizations are offering services to measure the relative effectiveness and efficiency of hospitals using the type of data listed in appendixes D through F. These organizations typically sell reports and studies to third-party payers and employers to be used in the managed care negotiating process. They also sell the studies to hospitals to be used in managed care negotiations as well as to compare a particular hospital operation to others. Although publicly available health care data do have many uses, they are inherently flawed with respect to measuring hospital efficiency and effectiveness.

Publicly available data are limited with respect to measuring hospital efficiency and effectiveness for the following reasons:

- *Claims data have errors and omissions:* Most of the data being analyzed are claims data from inpatient hospital discharge data tapes. Claims data are notoriously "dirty" with respect to accurately reflecting the resources used in a patient's care. For example:
  - Simple coding errors are legion.
  - Services for which there is no charge are missing entirely.
  - Claims data and service coding are manipulated to maximize reimbursement.
  - Claims data focus on charges that are largely meaningless because of the tremendous revenue deductions that are typically taken for hospital services. The most dramatic illustration of the irrelevancy of charges comes from the Financial Accounting Standards Board (FASB). This board sets accounting standards for all types of industry. Because of the magnitude of difference between gross charges and collections, FASB has directed hospitals to begin reporting only net revenue and to virtually ignore gross charges.
- *Effectiveness cannot be measured with claims data:* Effectiveness is measuring the result of applying a set of resources to achieve a certain end. In health care, outcomes measurement seems to be the most common way of assessing effectiveness. Except for using mortality rates, trying to determine medical outcomes from inpatient claims data is specious at best. Further, even if gross outcomes can be measured (for example, the patient died) using claims data, it is nigh well impossible to say whether those outcomes are within the expected range given the patient's underlying medical condition.
- *Data are only available for part of the care delivery process:* Another complication of using publicly available data to measure efficiency and effectiveness is that patients typically receive services from a broad selection of health care providers. Health care professional services are nearly always part of different systems or are independent entities. For example, physicians are usually part of a different economic entity than the hospital; the patient's home health service may be independent from both the hospital and physician group. The fragmented nature of the health care system means that data for the entire episode of care are scattered among a variety of independent entities. Further, most entities are not required to report data as hospitals are.

     The problem of reporting data from various services can be vexing even within a single hospital. For example, some hospitals have step-down units for orthopedic patients. The hospital splits the inpatient stay for a patient needing a hip replacement between the normal orthopedic unit and the step-down unit, which results in higher reimbursement from Medicare. Because of Medicare payment requirements, the patient is actually "discharged" from the hospital when he or she is transferred to the step-down unit, even though the patient will only be moved to another part of the hospital (sometimes just down the hall). If an uninformed observer compared data for hip replacements from a hospital with a step-down unit with data from a hospital that kept the patient on the orthopedic unit for the entire stay, the hospital with the step-down unit would appear to have a length of stay half the length of that of the traditional hospital! To illustrate the irony of this situation further, the patient in the step-down unit may end up staying longer than the patient in the traditional unit because rehabilitation usually starts in the step-down unit, whereas rehabilitation for the traditional service may be done by home health providers.

- *Medicare cost reports contain data that are not comparable:* Medicare cost reports are the other general source of data for organizations that provide efficiency and effectiveness analysis. As mentioned elsewhere in this book, Medicare cost reports are somewhat like tax returns in that there are strategies and tactics in completing them that can mean millions of dollars in additional revenue to a typical hospital. Another source of complication is that the organizations using cost reports to prepare efficiency and effectiveness studies assume that each hospital's cost structure and service structure is roughly comparable. This can be misleading; for example, university hospitals typically include the cost of clinics for outpatient care in their cost report. In many university hospitals, there are several hundred employees engaged in physician clinic operations that a typical community hospital would not have. The cost reports for these hospitals reflect the costs of the clinics, employees, supplies, and so forth, so overall cost measurements generally appear to be much higher than in a similarly sized community hospital.

- *Measurement of efficiency and effectiveness relies on severity adjustment:* Aside from addressing the other problems in this list, measures of effectiveness and efficiency should be done for similar patients. Measuring patient severity of illness is a notoriously tricky business that cannot be done using claims data. In fact, it may not be able to be done using medical records data as currently collected. For example, imagine trying to get comparable data for hip replacement patients: one would like to have quantitative measures of disability, pain, range of motion, and so forth before and after the replacement. This information simply is not collected consistently by health care providers.

Despite all of the foregoing limitations, the studies and reports, as they say, are "selling like hotcakes." This presents serious problems for many hospitals, particularly tertiary care facilities. Most payers do not understand the limitations of the data. To the extent that payers make managed care contracting decisions based on misunderstandings of the data's limitations, some hospitals could be severely hurt. Hospitals, particularly tertiary care facilities, must be ready to help educate payers and to respond with their own data regarding effectiveness and efficiency.

Monitoring the Political Process

Government's involvement in the health care sector has increased exponentially over the past 40 years, and it continues to grow. Gone forever are the days when decisions regarding health care were made solely by health care organizations, professionals, and patients. The nature of our system is being shaped by decisions made by Congress, state legislatures, and a number of regulatory agencies. Consequently, monitoring the political environment is critical.

Acquiring Political Information

Health care executives and managers can use two distinct approaches to obtain information about legislation being considered at the state and federal levels.

Knowing the Lobbyists

The first approach to obtaining information about legislation is to use the resources of state and national associations, such as state hospital associations and the American Hospital Association. These organizations employ professional lobbyists to monitor legislation and influence its development. In addition, most associations publish one or more newsletters on legislative developments. Professional lobbyists know which bills have a serious chance of being passed and at what stages in the legislative process a bill can be influenced.

In addition to reading legislative publications issued by associations, health care executives and managers may wish to become acquainted with association lobbyists. This is more easily done at the state level. Although lobbyists generally welcome the involvement and interest of association members, there are certain periods when legislative demands on their time are severe. Association members may need to be patient at such times.

Knowing the Legislators

The second approach to acquiring political information is to get to know the legislators. If they make the effort, health care executives and managers can become very well informed about what a legislature is doing. The key is to develop strong, personal relationships with state and federal legislators.

Three types of valuable political intelligence can be obtained through personal relationships with legislators. The first is advance notice of legislation still in development. Months before a bill is actually filed, one or more legislators will begin working on it. If health care executives and managers know their legislators well, they can be brought into the process at this stage. Knowing about legislation when it is first being developed is probably the most valuable type of political information that can be obtained.

The second type of political intelligence that can be obtained from personal relationships is information about what legislators are really thinking. Any reasonably astute observer of the political process soon realizes that legislators sometimes say one thing in public but think something quite different in private. A legislator can provide information about the private side of politics. (This, of course, is one big reason for the existence of professional lobbyists. They can find out what is being done in private.)

The third type of political intelligence is current information about what is happening to a bill while it is going through the legislative process. Knowing the status of a bill is useful because it can give health care managers a final chance to influence legislation.

Building Relationships with Elected Officials

If health care executives and managers wish to influence the legislative decisions that affect their institutions, they must become involved at the grassroots level. Understanding that politics is *local and personal* is the most important factor in influencing the political process.

Our legislative process operates as a highly competitive democracy influenced by special-interest groups. At both the federal and state levels, most legislative issues are decided on the basis of competition among those groups having the most at stake in the legislation under consideration. Whenever a piece of legislation is passed, some groups win and some groups lose. Most important, only those individuals and groups that actively compete in the political process will play a role in determining the ultimate outcome. Those who compete are *players* in the system; those who do not compete are *victims*. There is no middle ground.

The Local Nature of All Politics

For virtually all individuals working in the health care field, there are five key legislators whom they should know. At the federal level, two U.S. senators and one member of Congress represent each person in the United States. At the state level, that representation generally translates into one senator and one representative. This makes creating a personal relationship with politicians much simpler than it would appear. Health care executives need to focus their attention on those legislators who represent them. It is only the *local* representation that matters. Admittedly, a U.S. senator from California represents about 30 million people. This may not seem very local, but the principle still holds true, although the relationship may need to be established with a staff person rather than directly with the legislator.

The Personal Nature of All Politics

The next issue to be addressed is how those in the health care system can best make their views known. This chapter has already established that politics is not only local but also personal. Monitoring the political process will be easier if a personal relationship exists between constituents and legislators or their staff members. One of the best ways to facilitate a personal relationship is to provide legislators with factual information as well as perceptions and opinions.

Legislators at the federal and state levels deeply value input from their constituents. The question is how to best provide that input. It is important to realize three things. First, legislators deal with literally hundreds of issues. They cannot be equally well informed on all of them. Thus, legislators have a very real need for accurate, reliable information. Second, input can be provided more successfully if a constituent knows the legislator, the legislative process, and the issue. Third, like all human beings, legislators are more likely to respond if they are treated well. Showing concern about and interest in a legislator is essential if a constituent wants his or her views heard.

Campaigns and Personal Relationships

The best time for a constituent to build a strong, personal relationship with an individual running for a seat in the legislature is during the candidate's campaign for office. Assisting with a campaign generally provides access to the legislator and fosters his or her willingness to listen to opinions from his or her constituents after the election.

One of the least time-consuming and most obvious ways to help with a political campaign is by making a direct donation. Federal races are extremely expensive, and even state races cost a lot of money. There are federal limits on donations to candidates for the U.S. Senate and House of Representatives. The candidate's campaign office can provide information on these limits. Another source of information is state and national associations. Some states also may set limits on campaign donations.

Joining a political action committee is another easy step. Political action committees are associated with trade and professional organizations. Funds are pooled and donated to candidates. In this way, many small contributors can band together to increase their influence.

Volunteering to work on a campaign is another very effective means of involvement. Volunteering can include working on voter registration drives, telephone campaigns, and get-out-the-vote drives. Candidates never have enough time, money, or volunteers, but all are essential for a successful campaign.

Finally, one of the best ways to assist a candidate is to organize a fund-raising event. Fund-raisers can be held in private homes or, for more ambitious events, in hotels or other meeting places. Such events are particularly helpful because the work of planning and putting on the fund-raisers is done by individuals outside the campaign staff.

Communication of Constituent Views

Constituents can most effectively make their views known to their legislators, and thus influence the legislative process, if they heed the following advice:

- *Know the five key legislators who represent their institution.* It is essential to know each legislator's party as well as his or her profession, committee assignments, and past voting record. A call to the legislator's office usually brings more than enough information. Professional and trade associations usually employ government relations personnel who can offer important insights into the legislator's background, interests, and current work.
- *Know the legislative process.* At the federal level, knowing the process means being absolutely certain of committee assignments. Much of the actual development work for legislation in the U.S. Congress occurs in committees. State legislatures differ greatly in the importance and use of committees. Professional and trade associations can be very helpful in providing information about the legislative process.
- *Know the issue.* Any constituent providing information to a legislator must be absolutely sure that his or her facts are accurate. If there is proposed legislation, the constituent must know both what is and what is not contained in the bill.
- *Make use of staff.* Legislators, especially at the federal level, rely heavily on their staff. Those constituents who find it difficult to make direct personal contact with a U.S. senator or representative may find that contacting one of the legislator's staff members can facilitate access.

Building relationships with elected officials is important groundwork in the process of most effectively acquiring information about the politics affecting health care. Constituents will find their efforts rewarded if they follow a few simple rules: First, do not try to coerce legislators (for example, "If you don't vote the way we want you to, we'll make sure you're defeated in the next election"). Second, be prepared to answer legislators' questions. Finally, use appropriate protocol in all correspondence with legislators.

Conclusion

Gathering and analyzing appropriate information is an even more critical task as decision makers search for ways to make their institutions more responsive to the needs of the communities they seek to serve. However, those decision makers are faced with an enduring dilemma. On the one hand, decisions made without adequate information are inherently risky, although this approach does have the virtue of allowing decisions to be made rapidly. On the other hand, to indefinitely delay making decisions because of a lack of "perfect" information may be self-defeating and result in a lost opportunity.

Hospital administrators face an ever-increasing list of priorities, most of which require decisions having both short-and long-term consequences. In addition, many of the decisions—for example, the allocation of scarce capital among competing projects, the formulation of managed care strategies, and the expansion of patient care services—carry significantly higher risks today than they would have just a decade ago.

The strategy control system, data analysis techniques, sources of data, and bibliography of selected studies in this book are all tools to help health care managers anticipate and implement effective plans to seize opportunities and minimize the impact of environmental change. Essentially, the material in this book provides a foundation of information upon which decisions on specific issues can be based. To draw an analogy from nautical science, the application of these ideas may help the reader to identify the bearing and strength of the wind as well as to locate the shoreline, shoals, and reefs in hospital management decision making.

Appendix A

A Guide to Inpatient Data

Admission and Discharge Information

State	Total	Medical	Intensive Care Unit	Surgical	Obstetrics	Pediatrics	Neonatal
	Admission/Discharge Data Availability						
	General Medical/Surgical Units						
Alabama	X	X	X	X	X	X	X
Alaska	X	X	X	X	X	X	X
Arizona	X 0	X	X	X	X	X	X
Arkansas	X	X	X	X	X	X	X
California	X		X		X	X	X
Colorado	X 0	X	X	X	X	X	X
Connecticut	X 0	X 0	X 0	X 0	X 0	X 0	X 0
Delaware	X						
Florida	X	X	X	X	X	X	X
Georgia	X	X	X	X	X	X	X
Hawaii	X	X	X	X	X	X	X
Idaho	X	X	X	X	X	X	
Illinois	X	X	X	X	X	X	X
Indiana	X						
Iowa	X	X	X	X	X	X	X
Kansas	X						
Kentucky	X	X	X	X	X	X	X
Louisiana							
Maine	X						
Maryland	X	X	X	X	X	X	X
Massachusetts	X	X			X	X	
Michigan	X	X		X	X	X	X
Minnesota	X 0	X	X	X	X	X	X
Mississippi	X	X	X	X	X	X	X
Missouri	X	X	X	X	X	X	X
Montana							
Nebraska		X					X
Nevada	X	X	X	X	X	X	X
New Hampshire	X	X	X	X	X	X	X
New Jersey	X	X	X	X	X	X	X
New Mexico	X 0				0	0	0
New York[a]							
North Carolina	X	X	X	X	X	X	X
North Dakota	X	X		X	X	X	X
Ohio	X 0	X 0	X 0	X 0	X 0	X 0	X 0
Oklahoma							
Oregon	X	X	X	X	X	X	X
Pennsylvania	X	X	X		X	X	X
Rhode Island							
South Carolina	X	X	X	X	X	X	X
South Dakota	X	X	X	X	X	X	X
Tennessee	X 0	0	0	X 0	X 0	0	X 0
Texas	X	X	X	X	X	X	X
Utah	X	X	X	X	X	X	X
Vermont	X						
Virginia	X	X	X	X	X	X	X
Washington	X	X	X	X	X	X	X
West Virginia	X	X	X	X	X	X	X
Wisconsin[a]							
Wyoming	X 0	X 0	X 0	X 0	X 0	X 0	X 0

Note: X indicates data are available from a state facility, and 0 indicates data are available from a state hospital association.

[a]The states of New York and Wisconsin indicated that they collected and disseminated extensive utilization and financial information; however, neither state provided a breakdown of the specific information available.

Admission and Discharge Information (Continued)

State	Specialty Units — Psychiatric	Specialty Units — Rehabilitation	Extended Care — Skilled Nursing Facility	Extended Care — Intermediate Care Facility	Utilization Data from Medicare Cost Report	Page Number for Additional Information
Alabama	X	X	X	X	X	62
Alaska	X		X	X	X	63
Arizona	X	X			X	64–65
Arkansas	X	X	X	X	X	66
California	X	X	X	X	X	67–68
Colorado	X 0	X 0	X	X	X	69–70
Connecticut	X 0	X 0	0	0	X 0	71–72
Delaware	X	X	X	X	X	73
Florida	X 0		X 0	X	X	74–75
Georgia	X	X	X	X	X	76–77
Hawaii	X	X	X	X	X	78
Idaho	X	X			X	79
Illinois	X	X	X	X	X	80–81
Indiana					X	82
Iowa	X	X	X	X	X	83–84
Kansas					X	85
Kentucky	X	X			X	86–87
Louisiana					X	88
Maine					X	89
Maryland	X	X			X	90–91
Massachusetts	X	X	X	X	X	92–93
Michigan	X		X	X	X	94–95
Minnesota	X 0	X	0		X	96–97
Mississippi	X	X	X		X	98
Missouri	X	X	X	X	X	99
Montana					X	100
Nebraska	X	X			X	101
Nevada	X	X	X	X	X	102
New Hampshire	X	X	X	X	X	103–4
New Jersey	X	X	X	X	X	105–6
New Mexico	0	0			X	107–8
New York					X	109–10
North Carolina	X	X	X	X	X	111–12
North Dakota	X	X			X	113
Ohio	X	X	X	X	X 0	114
Oklahoma					X	115
Oregon	X	X	X	X	X	116
Pennsylvania		X	X	X	X	117–18
Rhode Island					X	119
South Carolina	X	X	X	X	X	120–21
South Dakota	X	X	X	X	X	122–23
Tennessee	X 0	0			X	124
Texas	X	X	X	X	X	125
Utah	X	X	X	X	X	126
Vermont					X	127–28
Virginia	X	X	X	X	X	129–30
Washington	X	X	X		X	131–32
West Virginia	X	X	X	X	X	133
Wisconsin					X	134–35
Wyoming	X 0	X 0	X 0	X 0	X	136

Note: X indicates data are available from a state facility, and 0 indicates data are available from a state hospital association.

Ancillary Services Information

State	Surgery	Number of Procedures/Visits				
		Diagnostic Radiology			Therapeutic Radiology	
		Magnetic Resonance Imaging	CT Scan	Radiology/ Fluoroscopy	Radiation Therapy	Radioactive Isotopes
Alabama	X	X	X			
Alaska		X	X		X	
Arizona	0					
Arkansas	X					
California	X				X	
Colorado	X 0	X	X	X	X	
Connecticut	X 0	X 0	X 0	X 0	X 0	X 0
Delaware	X	X	X	X	X	X
Florida		X	X		X	
Georgia	X	X	X		X	X
Hawaii		X	X		X	
Idaho	X	X	X	X	X	X
Illinois	X	X	X		X	
Indiana	X					
Iowa	X					
Kansas						
Kentucky	X	X	X			
Louisiana						
Maine	X	X	X			
Maryland	X	X	X	X	X	X
Massachusetts	X	X	X	X	X	X
Michigan	X	X	X	X	X	X
Minnesota	X	X	X		X	
Mississippi	X	X	X		X	X
Missouri	X	X	X			
Montana						
Nebraska	X	X	X		X	
Nevada	X	X	X		X	
New Hampshire	X	X	X	X	X	X
New Jersey		X	X			
New Mexico						
New York						
North Carolina	X	X	X	X	X	X
North Dakota						
Ohio	X	X	X	X	X	X
Oklahoma						
Oregon	X	X	X	X	X	X
Pennsylvania	X	X	X	X	X	X
Rhode Island						
South Carolina	X	X	X		X	X
South Dakota	X					
Tennessee	X 0	X	X		X 0	
Texas	X					
Utah	X	X	X	X	X	X
Vermont						
Virginia	X	X	X	X	X	X
Washington	X	X	X	X	X	
West Virginia	X	X	X	X	X	
Wisconsin						
Wyoming	X 0					

Note: X indicates data are available from a state facility, and 0 indicates data are available from a state hospital association.

Ancillary Services Information (Continued)

		Number of Procedures/Visits			
		Rehabilitation Services			
State	Laboratory	Physical Therapy	Occupational Therapy	Respiratory Therapy	Speech Therapy
Alabama					
Alaska		X			
Arizona					
Arkansas					
California					
Colorado					
Connecticut	X 0	X 0	X 0	X 0	X 0
Delaware	X	X	X	X	X
Florida					
Georgia	X	X			
Hawaii					
Idaho		X	X	X	X
Illinois					
Indiana					
Iowa					
Kansas					
Kentucky					
Louisiana					
Maine					
Maryland	X	X	X	X	X
Massachusetts	X	X	X	X	X
Michigan	X	X	X	X	X
Minnesota					
Mississippi		X	X		
Missouri					
Montana					
Nebraska					
Nevada	X	X	X		
New Hampshire		X	X	X	X
New Jersey					
New Mexico					
New York					
North Carolina	X	X	X	X	X
North Dakota					
Ohio	X	X	X	X	X
Oklahoma					
Oregon	X	X	X	X	X
Pennsylvania		X	X	X	X
Rhode Island					
South Carolina		X			
South Dakota					
Tennessee		X 0	X		X
Texas					
Utah	X	X	X	X	X
Vermont					
Virginia	X	X	X	X	X
Washington	X	X	X	X	X
West Virginia	X	X	X	X	X
Wisconsin					
Wyoming					

Note: X indicates data are available from a state facility, and 0 indicates data are available from a state hospital association.

Ancillary Services Information (Continued)

State	Nuclear Medicine	Open-Heart Surgeries	Cardiac Catheterizations	Stress Testing	Echocardiography
		Number of Procedures/Visits			
		Cardiology/Cardiac Surgery			
Alabama		X	X		
Alaska		X	X		
Arizona					
Arkansas					
California		X	X		
Colorado		X	X		
Connecticut	X O	X O	X O	X O	X O
Delaware					
Florida	X		X		
Georgia		X	X		
Hawaii	X				
Idaho		X	X		
Illinois		X	X		
Indiana		X	X		
Iowa					
Kansas					
Kentucky		X	X		
Louisiana					
Maine			X	X	
Maryland	X	X	X	X	X
Massachusetts	X	X	X	X	X
Michigan	X	X	X		
Minnesota		X	X		
Mississippi	X	X	X		
Missouri		X	X		
Montana					
Nebraska		X	X		
Nevada		X	X		
New Hampshire	X	X	X		
New Jersey	X	X	X		
New Mexico					
New York					
North Carolina	X	X	X	X	X
North Dakota					
Ohio		X	X		
Oklahoma					
Oregon	X	X	X	X	X
Pennsylvania	X	X	X		
Rhode Island					
South Carolina		X	X		
South Dakota					
Tennessee	X O	X O	X O		
Texas					
Utah	X	X	X		X
Vermont					
Virginia	X	X	X		
Washington	X				
West Virginia	X	X	X		
Wisconsin					
Wyoming		X			

Note: X indicates data are available from a state facility, and 0 indicates data are available from a state hospital association.

Ancillary Services Information (Continued)

State	Number of Procedures/Visits Cardiology/Cardiac Surgery		Information from Medicare Cost Report	Page Number for Additional Information
	Electrocardiography	Electroencephalograpy		
Alabama			X	62
Alaska			X	63
Arizona			X	64–65
Arkansas			X	66
California			X	67–68
Colorado			X	69–70
Connecticut	X 0	X 0	X	71–72
Delaware	X	X	X	73
Florida			X	74–75
Georgia			X	76–77
Hawaii			X	78
Idaho		X	X	79
Illinois			X	80–81
Indiana			X	82
Iowa			X	83–84
Kansas			X	85
Kentucky			X	86–87
Louisiana			X	88
Maine			X	89
Maryland	X	X	X	90–91
Massachusetts	X	X	X	92–93
Michigan	X	X	X	94–95
Minnesota			X	96–97
Mississippi			X	98
Missouri			X	99
Montana			X	100
Nebraska			X	101
Nevada			X	102
New Hampshire			X	103–4
New Jersey			X	105–6
New Mexico			X	107–8
New York			X	109–10
North Carolina	X	X	X	111–12
North Dakota			X	113
Ohio			X 0	114
Oklahoma			X	115
Oregon			X	116
Pennsylvania			X	117–18
Rhode Island			X	119
South Carolina			X	120–21
South Dakota			X	122–23
Tennessee			X	124
Texas			X	125
Utah	X	X	X	126
Vermont			X	127–28
Virginia			X	129–30
Washington			X	131–32
West Virginia	X	X	X	133
Wisconsin				134–35
Wyoming			X	136

Note: X indicates data are available from a state facility, and 0 indicates data are available from a state hospital association.

Appendix B

A Guide to Outpatient Data

Procedure and Visit Information

State	Emergency Room	Ambulatory Surgery	Magnetic Resonance Imaging	CT Scan	Radiology/ Fluoroscopy
			Number of Procedures/Visits		
			Outpatient Diagnostic Radiology		
Alabama	X		X	X	
Alaska	X				
Arizona	0	0			
Arkansas	X				
California	X				
Colorado	X 0	X 0	X	X	
Connecticut	X 0	X 0			
Delaware					
Florida					
Georgia	X	X			
Hawaii				X	
Idaho	X	X	X	X	
Illinois			X	X	
Indiana	X		X	X	
Iowa	X				
Kansas	X				
Kentucky	X	X	X	X	
Louisiana					
Maine		X			
Maryland		X			
Massachusetts	X	X	X	X	X
Michigan	X	X	X	X	X
Minnesota	X 0	X	X		
Mississippi	X	X	X		X
Missouri	X	X	X	X	
Montana					
Nebraska	X	X	X	X	
Nevada	X	X	X	X	
New Hampshire	X	X	X		
New Jersey	X	X	X	X	X
New Mexico	0	0			
New York[a]					
North Carolina	X	X	X	X	X
North Dakota					
Ohio	X		X	X	X
Oklahoma					
Oregon	X	X	X	X	X
Pennsylvania	X	X	X	X	X
Rhode Island					
South Carolina	X	X	X	X	
South Dakota	X	X			
Tennessee	X 0	X 0	X	X	
Texas	X				
Utah	X		X	X	X
Vermont		X			
Virginia	X	X	X	X	X
Washington	X	X			
West Virginia	X	X	X	X	
Wisconsin[a]					
Wyoming	X 0	X 0			

Note: X indicates data are available from a state facility, and 0 indicates data are available from a state hospital association.

[a]The states of New York and Wisconsin indicated that they collected and disseminated extensive utilization and financial information; however, neither state provided a breakdown of the specific information available.

Procedure and Visit Information (Continued)

	Number of Procedures/Visits						
	Outpatient Therapeutic Radiology		Outpatient Lab	Outpatient Rehabilitation Services			
State	Radiation Therapy	Radioactive Isotopes		Physical Therapy	Occupational Therapy	Respiratory Therapy	Speech Therapy
Alabama							
Alaska							
Arizona							
Arkansas							
California							
Colorado							
Connecticut	0	0	0	0	0	0	0
Delaware							
Florida							
Georgia							
Hawaii							
Idaho							
Illinois							
Indiana							
Iowa							
Kansas							
Kentucky							
Louisiana							
Maine							
Maryland							
Massachusetts	X	X	X	X	X	X	X
Michigan	X	X		X	X	X	X
Minnesota							
Mississippi	X			X	X		
Missouri							
Montana							
Nebraska	X						
Nevada	X						
New Hampshire							
New Jersey							
New Mexico							
New York							
North Carolina	X	X					
North Dakota							
Ohio	X	X	X				
Oklahoma							
Oregon	X	X	X	X	X	X	X
Pennsylvania	X	X		X	X	X	X
Rhode Island							
South Carolina	X			X			
South Dakota							
Tennessee	X			X	X		X
Texas							
Utah	X	X	X	X	X	X	X
Vermont							
Virginia	X						
Washington							
West Virginia	X						
Wisconsin							
Wyoming							

Note: X indicates data are available from a state facility, and 0 indicates data are available from a state hospital association.

Procedure and Visit Information (Continued)

| State | Outpatient Nuclear Medicine | Outpatient Cardiology | | | Outpatient Electrocardiography | Outpatient Electroencephalography | Page Number for Additional Information |
		Cardiac Catheterizations	Stress Testing	Echocardiography			
Alabama							62
Alaska							63
Arizona							64-65
Arkansas							66
California							67-68
Colorado		X					69-70
Connecticut	0	0	0	0	0	0	71-72
Delaware							73
Florida							74-75
Georgia							76-77
Hawaii							78
Idaho		X					79
Illinois							80-81
Indiana		X					82
Iowa							83-84
Kansas							85
Kentucky		X	X				86-87
Louisiana							88
Maine		X	X				89
Maryland							90-91
Massachusetts	X	X	X	X	X	X	92-93
Michigan							94-95

State					Page
Minnesota					96-97
Mississippi					98
Missouri					99
Montana					100
Nebraska	X				101
Nevada	X				102
New Hampshire					103-4
New Jersey	X				105-6
New Mexico					107-8
New York					109-10
North Carolina	X				111-12
North Dakota					113
Ohio	X				114
Oklahoma					115
Oregon	X	X	X	X	116
Pennsylvania	X				117-18
Rhode Island					119
South Carolina	X				120-21
South Dakota					122-23
Tennessee	X 0				124
Texas		X			125
Utah	X		X	X	126
Vermont					127-28
Virginia	X				129-30
Washington					131-32
West Virginia	X				133
Wisconsin					134-35
Wyoming					136

Note: X indicates data are available from a state facility, and 0 indicates data are available from a state hospital association.

Appendix C

A Guide to Financial Data

Income Statement Information

State	Gross Revenue	Revenue Deductions	Net Revenue	Gross by Department/ Service	Net by Department/ Service
	Revenue Data				
Alabama					
Alaska					
Arizona	X 0	X 0	X 0		
Arkansas					
California	X	X	X	X	X
Colorado	X 0	X 0	X 0		
Connecticut	X 0	X 0	X 0	X 0	X 0
Delaware					
Florida	X	X	X	X	
Georgia	X	X	X		
Hawaii					
Idaho					
Illinois					
Indiana	X	X	X	X	X
Iowa					
Kansas	X				
Kentucky					
Louisiana					
Maine	X				
Maryland	X	X	X	X	X
Massachusetts	X	X	X		
Michigan					
Minnesota	X 0	0	0		
Mississippi					
Missouri	X	X	X		
Montana					
Nebraska					
Nevada	X	X	X	X	
New Hampshire	X	X	X		
New Jersey					
New Mexico					
New York[a]					
North Carolina					
North Dakota					
Ohio	0	0	0	0	0
Oklahoma					
Oregon	X	X	X	X	X
Pennsylvania					
Rhode Island					
South Carolina	X	X	X		
South Dakota	X 0	X 0	X 0		
Tennessee	X 0	X	X 0		
Texas	X	X	X		
Utah	X		X		
Vermont	X				
Virginia	X 0	X 0	X 0		
Washington	X	X	X	X	X
West Virginia	X	X	X	X	
Wisconsin[a]					
Wyoming	X 0	X 0	X 0	X	X

Note: X indicates data are available from a state facility, and 0 indicates data are available from a state hospital association.
[a]The states of New York and Wisconsin indicated that they collected and disseminated extensive utilization and financial information; however, neither state provided a breakdown of the specific information available.

Income Statement Information (Continued)

State	Total Facility	Specific Department/ Service	Units of Service
		Revenue Data Available	
Alabama			
Alaska			
Arizona	X 0		
Arkansas			
California	X	X	X
Colorado	X 0		
Connecticut	X 0	X 0	0
Delaware			
Florida	X		
Georgia	X		
Hawaii			
Idaho			
Illinois			
Indiana	X	X	X
Iowa			
Kansas	X		
Kentucky			
Louisiana			
Maine	X		
Maryland	X	X	X
Massachusetts	X		
Michigan			
Minnesota	X 0		
Mississippi			
Missouri	X		
Montana			
Nebraska			
Nevada	X	X	
New Hampshire	X		
New Jersey			
New Mexico			
New York			
North Carolina			
North Dakota			
Ohio	0	0	0
Oklahoma			
Oregon	X	X	X
Pennsylvania			
Rhode Island			
South Carolina	X		
South Dakota	X 0		
Tennessee	X 0		
Texas	X		
Utah	X		
Vermont	X		
Virginia	X 0		X
Washington	X	X	X
West Virginia	X		X
Wisconsin			
Wyoming	X 0	X	X

Note: X indicates data are available from a state facility, and 0 indicates data are available from a state hospital association.

Income Statement Information (Continued)

State	Expense Data					Expense Detail Available			
	Total Expense	Total Direct Expense	Total Indirect Expense	Specific Direct Expense	Specific Indirect Expense	Total Facility	Direct by Department/Service	Indirect by Department/Service	Units of Service
Alabama	X								
Alaska									
Arizona	X 0					X 0			
Arkansas	X								
California	X	X	X	X	X	X	X	X	X
Colorado	X 0								
Connecticut	X 0	X 0	X 0	X 0	X 0	X 0	X 0	X 0	
Delaware									
Florida	X			X	X				
Georgia	X								
Hawaii									
Idaho									
Illinois									
Indiana	X	X	X	X	X	X	X	X	X
Iowa	X								
Kansas	X								
Kentucky									
Louisiana									
Maine	X								
Maryland	X	X	X	X	X	X	X	X	X
Massachusetts	X					X			
Michigan	X								

State	1	2	3	4	5	6	7	8	9
Minnesota	X O	O		O		O			
Mississippi	X								
Missouri						X			
Montana									
Nebraska									
Nevada	X	X	X		X	X			
New Hampshire	X	X	X						
New Jersey									
New Mexico									
New York									
North Carolina									
North Dakota									
Ohio	O	O	O	O	O	O	O	O	O
Oklahoma									
Oregon	X	X	X	X	X	X	X	X	X
Pennsylvania	X	X							
Rhode Island									
South Carolina	X								
South Dakota	X O	O				O			
Tennessee	X O	O				O			
Texas	X					X			
Utah	X								
Vermont	X								
Virginia	X O	X	X						X
Washington	X	X	X	X	X	X	X	X	X
West Virginia	X	X	X	X	X	X		X	X
Wisconsin									
Wyoming	X O	X O	X	X	X	X O			

Note: X indicates data are available from a state facility, and O indicates data are available from a state hospital association.

Income Statement Information (Continued)

State	Availability of Inpatient and Outpatient Data		Financial Data from Medicare Cost Reports	Page Number for Additional Information
	Inpatient	Outpatient		
Alabama			X	62
Alaska			X	63
Arizona			X	64–65
Arkansas			X	66
California			X	67–68
Colorado	X 0	X 0	X	69–70
Connecticut	0	0	X 0	71–72
Delaware	X		X	73
Florida	X	X	X	74–75
Georgia			X	76–77
Hawaii			X	78
Idaho			X	79
Illinois			X	80–81
Indiana			X	82
Iowa			X	83–84
Kansas			X	85
Kentucky			X	86–87
Louisiana			X	88
Maine			X	89
Maryland	X	X	X	90–91
Massachusetts	X		X	92–93
Michigan			X	94–95
Minnesota			X	96–97
Mississippi			X	98
Missouri	X	X	X	99
Montana			X	100
Nebraska			X	101
Nevada	X	X	X	102
New Hampshire			X	103–4
New Jersey			X	105–6
New Mexico			X	107–8
New York			X	109–10
North Carolina			X	111–12
North Dakota			X	113
Ohio	X		X 0	114
Oklahoma			X	115
Oregon	X	X	X	116
Pennsylvania			X	117–18
Rhode Island			X	119
South Carolina	X	X	X	120–21
South Dakota	X 0	X 0	X	122–23
Tennessee	X 0	X 0	X	124
Texas	X	X	X	125
Utah	X	X	X	126
Vermont			X	127–28
Virginia	X	X	X	129–30
Washington	X	X	X	131–32
West Virginia	X	X	X	133
Wisconsin			X	134–35
Wyoming	X	X	X 0	136

Note: X indicates data are available from a state facility, and 0 indicates data are available from a state hospital association.

Appendix D

Sources of Information, by State

Alabama

In addition to the data listed in appendixes A–C, the state of Alabama conducts a Patient Origin Study of April Discharges. Although data are not available by either DRG or ICD-9 code, they are arrayed in nine clinical service codes. All information is available on paper; discharges by clinical service code are also available on either tape or diskette. Charges vary according to the report and format. The state also collects data on the following specialty hospitals: psychiatric, children's, and rehabilitation.

Requests for data should be directed to:

Sherrie A. Cook, Director
Division of Data Management
State Health Planning and Development Agency
312 Montgomery Street, 7th Floor
Montgomery, AL 36104
(205) 242-4103 phone
(205) 242-4113 fax

Medicare cost reports can be requested from:

Provider Reimbursement
Blue Cross and Blue Shield of Alabama
450 Riverchase Parkway East
Birmingham, AL 35298
(205) 988-2733 phone
(205) 733-7419 fax

The state's hospital association can be contacted at:

Alabama Hospital Association
P.O. Box 210759
Montgomery, AL 36121-0759
(205) 272-8781 phone
(205) 270-9527 fax

The state's insurance commissioner can be contacted at:

State Insurance Commissioner
James H. Dill
Department of Insurance
State of Alabama
P.O. Box 303351
Montgomery, AL 36130-3351
(205) 269-3550 phone
(205) 269-3213 fax

Contact for health insurance information:
Harland Dyer
(205) 269-3202 phone

Contact for annual statement information:
Ann Strickland
(205) 269-3565 phone

Please note: Before data are requested from any source, it is advisable to telephone the source to confirm that the data sought are available in the time period desired. In addition, the cost and exact procedure for obtaining data are most easily explained in a telephone conversation.

Alaska

All data reporting in Alaska is on a voluntary basis. Inpatient data are available by ICD-9 code, on paper, and are $7.00 per copy. The latest data available are for 1991.

Requests for data should be directed to:

Robert Sylvester, Research Analyst
Planning Section
State of Alaska—Department of Health and Social Services
Division of Administrative Services
P.O. Box 110650
Juneau, AK 99811-0650
(907) 465-3082 phone
(907) 465-2499 fax

Medicare cost reports can be requested from:

Blue Cross of Washington and Alaska
P.O. Box 327
Mountlake Terrace, WA 98043
(800) 213-5470 phone
(206) 361-3198 fax

The state's hospital association can be contacted at:

Alaska State Hospital and Nursing Home Association
319 Seward Street, Suite 11
Juneau, AK 99801
(907) 586-1790 phone
(907) 463-3573 fax

The state's insurance commissioner can be contacted at:

State Insurance Commissioner
David J. Walsh
State of Alaska/Dept. of Commerce & Economic Development
Division of Insurance
P.O. Box 110805
Juneau, AK 99811-0805
(907) 465-2515 phone
(907) 465-3422 fax

Contact for health insurance information:
Thelma Walker (Anchorage)
(907) 349-1230 phone

Contact for annual statement information:
Dean George (Juneau)
(907) 465-4608 phone

Please note: Before data are requested from any source, it is advisable to telephone the source to confirm that the data sought are available in the time period desired. In addition, the cost and exact procedure for obtaining data are most easily explained in a telephone conversation.

Arizona

Discharge data for all hospitals with more than 50 beds are collected and available on either tape or diskette (effective January 1, 1995, data are available for all hospitals except psychiatric and substance abuse). Hospitals must also submit the following annually: (1) audited financial statements, (2) annual uniform accounting report, and (3) a copy of their Medicare Cost Report. Additionally, all hospitals, nursing care institutions, and outpatient treatment centers must file their rates and charges with the Department of Health Services.

Arizona participates in an Agency for Health Care Policy and Research project called the Healthcare Cost and Utilization Project (HCUP-3). HCUP-3 has created the State Inpatient Database, which provides comparable inpatient data for 12 states: Arizona, California, Colorado, Florida, Illinois, Iowa, Massachusetts, New Jersey, New York, Pennsylvania, Washington, and Wisconsin. Each state has established policies and procedures for gaining access to state data. Requests related to the Arizona HCUP-3 State Inpatient Database, and requests for other types of data, should be directed to:

Joe Brennan
Arizona Department of Health Services
Office of Health Planning, Evaluation, and Statistics
Cost Reporting and Review Section
1651 East Morton, Suite 110
Phoenix, AZ 85020
(602) 255-1140 phone
(602) 255-1135 fax

If information is needed regarding the HCUP-3 project in general, please contact the Agency for Health Care Policy and Research, Division of Provider Studies, Center for Intramural Research, (301) 594-1410 (phone), (301) 594-2314 (fax), hcupSID@cghsir.ahcpr.gov (via Internet).

Medicare cost reports can be requested from:

Blue Cross and Blue Shield of Arizona, Inc.
P.O. Box 13466
Phoenix, AZ 85002-3466
(602) 864-4298 phone
(602) 864-4062 fax

The state's hospital association can be contacted at:

Arizona Hospital Association
1501 West Fountainhead Parkway, Suite 650
Tempe, AZ 85282
(602) 968-1083 phone
(602) 967-2029 fax

The state's insurance commissioner can be contacted at:

State Insurance Commissioner
Chris Herstam
State of Arizona
Department of Insurance
2910 North 44th Street, Suite 210
Phoenix, AZ 85018-7256
(602) 912-8400 phone
(602) 912-8421 fax

Contact for health insurance information:
Shirley Polzin
(602) 912-8460 phone

Contact for annual statement information:
Barbara Lewis
(602) 912-8420 phone

Please note: Before data are requested from any source, it is advisable to telephone the source to confirm that the data sought are available in the time period desired. In addition, the cost and exact procedure for obtaining data are most easily explained in a telephone conversation.

Arkansas

No utilization or financial data are available. Medicare cost reports can be requested from:

Arkansas Blue Cross and Blue Shield, Inc.
601 Gaines Street
Little Rock, AR 72201
(501) 378-2248 phone
(501) 378-3040 fax

The state's hospital association can be contacted at:

Arkansas Hospital Association
419 Natural Resources Drive
Little Rock, AR 72205
(501) 224-7878 phone
(501) 224-0519 fax

The state's insurance commissioner can be contacted at:

State Insurance Commissioner
Lee Douglas
1123 South University Avenue, Suite 400
University Tower Building
Little Rock, AR 72204-1699
(501) 686-2900 phone
(501) 686-2913 fax

Contact for health insurance information:
John Shields
(501) 686-2875 phone

Contact for annual statement information:
Lewis Wharff
(501) 686-2855 phone

Please note: Before data are requested from any source, it is advisable to telephone the source to confirm that the data sought are available in the time period desired. In addition, the cost and exact procedure for obtaining data are most easily explained in a telephone conversation.

California

California maintains eight databases: *Financial:* Hospital Annual, Hospital Quarterly, Long-Term Care Annual; *Utilization:* Hospital, Home Health Agencies, Licensed Clinics, Long-Term Care; *Patient Discharge Data:* Patient Discharge Data. Data are available on paper, magnetic tape, or diskette. The charge varies according to the data requested.

California also participates in an Agency for Health Care Policy and Research project called the Healthcare Cost and Utilization Project (HCUP-3). HCUP-3 has created the State Inpatient Database, which provides comparable inpatient data for 12 states: Arizona, California, Colorado, Florida, Illinois, Iowa, Massachusetts, New Jersey, New York, Pennsylvania, Washington, and Wisconsin. Each state has established policies and procedures for gaining access to state data. Requests related to the California HCUP-3 State Inpatient Database should be directed to:

Kathy McCaffrey
California Office of Statewide Health Planning and Development
Health Facility Data Division
818 K Street, Room 500
Sacramento, CA 95814
(916) 323-8399 phone
(916) 324-9242 fax

If information is needed regarding the HCUP-3 project in general, please contact the Agency for Health Care Policy and Research, Division of Provider Studies, Center for Intramural Research, (301) 594-1410 (phone), (301) 594-2314 (fax), hcupSID@cghsir.ahcpr.gov (via Internet).

Other requests for data should be directed to:

Homero Lomas, Manager
California Office of Statewide Health Planning and Development
Data Users Support Group
818 K Street, Suite 500
Sacramento, CA 95814
(916) 322-2814 phone
(916) 324-9242 fax

Medicare cost reports can be requested from:

Blue Cross of California—Medicare
P.O. Box 70000
Van Nuys, CA 91470
(818) 593-2006 phone
(818) 703-2848 fax

The state's hospital association can be contacted at:

California Association of Hospitals and Health Systems
P.O. Box 1100
Sacramento, CA 95812-1100
(916) 443-7401 phone
(916) 552-7596 fax

The state's insurance commissioner can be contacted at:

State Insurance Commissioner
John Garmendi
State of California
Department of Insurance
770 L Street, Suite 1120
Sacramento, CA 95814
(916) 445-5544 phone
(916) 445-5280 fax

Contact for health insurance information:
Laura Rosenthal
(916) 322-9230 phone

Contact for annual statement information:
M. Elsa Enciso
(213) 346-6444 phone

Please note: Before data are requested from any source, it is advisable to telephone the source to confirm that the data sought are available in the time period desired. In addition, the cost and exact procedure for obtaining data are most easily explained in a telephone conversation.

Colorado

Colorado inpatient hospital data are available on paper only. Data are available by DRG and ICD-9 code.

Colorado participates in an Agency for Health Care Policy and Research project called the Healthcare Cost and Utilization Project (HCUP-3). HCUP-3 has created the State Inpatient Database, which provides comparable inpatient data for 12 states: Arizona, California, Colorado, Florida, Illinois, Iowa, Massachusetts, New Jersey, New York, Pennsylvania, Washington, and Wisconsin. Each state has established policies and procedures for gaining access to state data. Requests related to the Colorado HCUP-3 State Inpatient Database should be directed to:

Michael Boyson
Data Services Research
Colorado Hospital Association
2140 South Holly Street
Denver, CO 80222-5607
(303) 758-1630 phone
(303) 758-0047 fax

If information is needed regarding the HCUP-3 project in general, please contact the Agency for Health Care Policy and Research, Division of Provider Studies, Center for Intramural Research, (301) 594-1410 (phone), (301) 594-2314 (fax), hcupSID@cghsir.ahcpr.gov (via Internet).

Requests for hospital-level data should be directed to:

Reid Reynolds
Manager
Health Data Commission
Colorado Department of Health Care
   Policy and Financing
1575 Sherman Street, Room 418
Denver, CO 80203
(303) 866-2158 phone
(303) 866-2803 fax

Other requests for data should be directed to:

Sue E. Rehak
Colorado Health and Environmental Department
4300 Cherry Creek Drive South, HFD-A2
Denver, CO 80222-1530
(303) 692-2000 phone
(303) 782-4883 fax

Medicare cost reports can be requested from:

Peggy Franks
Blue Cross and Blue Shield of Colorado
Provider Audit Department, 8th Floor
700 Broadway
Denver, CO 80273
(303) 831-2798 phone
(303) 831-2012 fax

The state's hospital association can be contacted at:

Colorado Hospital Association
2140 South Holly Street
Denver, CO 80222-5607
(303) 758-1630 phone
(303) 758-0047 fax

Data contact person:

Michael Boyson
Director of Data Services
Colorado Hospital Association
2140 South Holly Street
Denver, CO 80222-5607
(303) 758-1630 phone
(303) 758-0047 fax

Data are available sorted by DRG and ICD-9 code on paper, magnetic tape, or diskette. The charge varies according to the data requested. Call for a price.

The state's insurance commissioner can be contacted at:

State Insurance Commissioner
Jack Ehnes
Colorado Division of Insurance
Colorado Department of Regulatory Agencies
1560 Broadway, Suite 850
Denver, CO 80202
(303) 894-7499 phone
(303) 894-7455 fax

Contact for health insurance information:
Barbara Yondorf
(303) 894-7499 ext. 308 phone

Contact for annual statement information:
Chad Collier
(303) 894-7499 ext. 323 phone

Please note: Before data are requested from any source, it is advisable to telephone the source to confirm that the data sought are available in the time period desired. In addition, the cost and exact procedure for obtaining data are most easily explained in a telephone conversation.

Connecticut

Connecticut data are available on paper, tape, or diskette. Data are sorted by DRG and ICD-9 code.

Requests for hospital-level data should be directed to:

Michael Hofmann
Senior Research Analyst
Connecticut Office of Health Care Access
1049 Asylum Avenue
Hartford, CT 06105-2431
(203) 566-7793 phone
(203) 566-5663 fax

Other requests for data should be directed to:

Joan Foland
Associate Research Analyst
Connecticut Office of Health Care Access
1049 Asylum Avenue
Hartford, CT 06105-2431
(203) 566-3880 phone
(203) 566-5663 fax

The state Medicare intermediary is:

Blue Cross and Blue Shield of Connecticut
370 Bassett Road
North Haven, CT 06473
(203) 630-4970 phone
(203) 630-4980 fax

The state's hospital association can be contacted at:

Connecticut Hospital Association
110 Barnes Road
P.O. Box 90
Wallingford, CT 06492-0090
(203) 265-7611 (phone)
(203) 284-9318 (fax)

Data contact persons:

Judy Marchione
110 Barnes Road
Wallingford, CT 06492

John Lynch, Vice-President, Research
Connecticut Hospital Association
P.O. Box 90
Wallingford, CT 06492-0090

Data are available by DRG or ICD-9 code in various formats. The charge varies according to the data requested.

The state's insurance commissioner can be contacted at:

Acting State Insurance Commissioner
William J. Gilligan
Department of Insurance
State of Connecticut
P.O. Box 816
Hartford, CT 06142-0816
(203) 297-3802 phone
(203) 566-7410 fax

Contact for health insurance information:
Allan B. Roby, Jr.
(203) 297-3862 phone

Contact for annual statement information:
Louis Scotti
(203) 297-3818 phone

Please note: Before data are requested from any source, it is advisable to telephone the source to confirm that the data sought are available in the time period desired. In addition, the cost and exact procedure for obtaining data are most easily explained in a telephone conversation.

Delaware

Delaware collects a variety of hospital data. In addition to hospital data, skilled nursing home and intermediate care facility utilization data are also available. Data are available by DRG and ICD-9 code on paper, tape, or floppy disk. The charge varies according to the data requested.

Requests for data should be directed to:

Donald L. Berry
Manager, Health Statistics and Research
Delaware Department of Health and Social Services
Bureau of Health Planning and Resources Management
P.O. Box 637
Dover, DE 19903
(302) 739-4776 phone
(302) 739-3008 fax

Medicare cost reports can be requested from:

Blue Cross and Blue Shield of Delaware, Inc.
P.O. Box 1991
Wilmington, DE 19899
(302) 429-0260 phone
(302) 421-2060 fax

The state's hospital association can be contacted at:

Association of Delaware Hospitals
1280 South Governors Avenue
Dover, DE 19904-4802
(302) 674-2853 phone
(302) 734-2731 fax

The state's insurance commissioner can be contacted at:

State Insurance Commissioner
Donna Lee Williams
Department of Insurance
State of Delaware
Rodney Building, 841 Silver Lake Boulevard
Dover, DE 19904
(302) 739-4251 phone
(302) 739-5280 fax

Contact for health insurance information:
Marianne Chillas
(302) 739-4251 phone

Contact for annual statement information:
Steven White
(302) 739-4251 ext. 41 phone

Please note: Before data are requested from any source, it is advisable to telephone the source to confirm that the data sought are available in the time period desired. In addition, the cost and exact procedure for obtaining data are most easily explained in a telephone conversation.

Florida

The Agency for Health Care Administration provides a catalog of the data available from the Agency health care databases. The data are divided into the following categories:

- Ambulatory and other data
- Hospital patient and financial data
- Nursing home patient and financial data
- Psychiatric patient and financial data
- Publications and studies

Data are available variously on paper, diskette, and magnetic tape. Call or write for the prices of specific items.

Florida participates in an Agency for Health Care Policy and Research project called the Healthcare Cost and Utilization Project (HCUP-3). HCUP-3 has created the State Inpatient Database, which provides comparable inpatient data for 12 states: Arizona, California, Colorado, Florida, Illinois, Iowa, Massachusetts, New Jersey, New York, Pennsylvania, Washington, and Wisconsin. Each state has established policies and procedures for gaining access to state data. Requests related to the Florida HCUP-3 State Inpatient Database should be directed to:

Randy Mutter
Florida Agency for Health Care Administration
State Center for Health Statistics
Research and Analysis Section
325 John Knox Road, Suite 301
The Atrium
Tallahassee, FL 32303
(904) 922-5572 phone
(904) 921-0973 fax
rmutter@wane.leon.mail via Internet

If information is needed regarding the HCUP-3 project in general, please contact the Agency for Health Care Policy and Research, Division of Provider Studies, Center for Intramural Research, (301) 594-1410 (phone), (301) 594-2314 (fax), hcupSID@cghsir.ahcpr.gov (via Internet).

Other requests for data should be directed to:

State of Florida
Ron Lawrence, Research Associate, Special Reports and Analysis
Florida Agency for Health Care Administration
State Center for Health Statistics
Research and Analysis Section
2727 Mahan Drive
Building 1, Room 301A
Tallahassee, FL 32308-5403
(904) 921-0550 phone
(904) 922-6964 fax

Medicare cost reports can be requested from:

Provider Audit and Reimbursement Department
Blue Cross and Blue Shield of Florida, Inc.
P.O. Box 45268
Jacksonville, FL 32232-5268
(904) 791-8570 phone
(904) 791-8441 fax

The state's hospital association can be contacted at:

Florida Hospital Association
P.O. Box 531107
Orlando, FL 32853-1107
(407) 841-6230 phone
(407) 422-5948 fax

Data contact person:

Kim Streit
Florida Hospital Association
P.O. Box 531107
Orlando, FL 32853-1107
(407) 841-6230 phone

Data are available by DRG code on magnetic tape or diskette. The charge varies according to the data requested.

The state's insurance commissioner can be contacted at:

State Insurance Commissioner
Bill Nelson
Department of Insurance/State Treasurer's Office
State of Florida
State Capitol/Plaza Level Eleven
Tallahassee, FL 32399-0300
(904) 922 3100 phone
(904) 488-3334 fax

Contact for health insurance information:
Tom Foley
(904) 922-3152 phone

Contact for annual statement information:
John Black
(904) 922-3153 phone

Please note: Before data are requested from any source, it is advisable to telephone the source to confirm that the data sought are available in the time period desired. In addition, the cost and exact procedure for obtaining data are most easily explained in a telephone conversation.

Georgia

Georgia collects data from hospitals, ambulatory surgery centers, and skilled nursing facilities. Data are available either on paper or floppy disk. The charge varies according to the data requested.

Requests for hospital-level data should be directed to:

Jim Griffin
Director
Health Assessment Services
Georgia Public Health Services
2 Peachtree Street, NW
3rd Floor, Annex
Atlanta, GA 30303
(404) 657-6326 phone
(404) 657-6282 fax

Other requests for data should be directed to:

Lucille Brookshaw, Director
Program Support Division
State Health Planning Agency
4 Executive Park Drive NE, Suite 2100
Atlanta, GA 30329
(404) 679-4833 phone
(404) 679-4914 fax

Medicare cost reports can be requested from:

Blue Cross and Blue Shield of Georgia—Medicare
P.O. Box 9048
Columbus, GA 31908-9048
(706) 322-4082 phone
(706) 571-5431 fax

The state's hospital association can be contacted at:

Georgia Hospital Association
1675 Terrell Mill Road
Marietta, GA 30067
(404) 955-0324 phone
(404) 955-5801 fax

The state's insurance commissioner can be contacted at:

State Insurance Commissioner
Tim Ryles
Department of Insurance/State of Georgia
2 Martin Luther King, Jr. Dr./Floyd Memorial Building
704 West Tower
Atlanta, GA 30334
(404) 656-2056 phone
(404) 657-9831 fax

Contact for health insurance information:
Stan Miller
(404) 656-2085 phone

Contact for annual statement information:
Tom Carswell
(404) 656-2074 phone

Please note: Before data are requested from any source, it is advisable to telephone the source to confirm that the data sought are available in the time period desired. In addition, the cost and exact procedure for obtaining data are most easily explained in a telephone conversation.

Hawaii

Hawaii data are available on paper only. Requests for data should be directed to:

Ken Yoshida, Statistician
State Health Planning and Development Agency
335 Merchant Street, Suite 214E
Honolulu, HI 96813
(808) 587-0788 phone
(808) 587-0783 fax

Medicare cost reports can be requested from:

Winnie Odo, Administrator
Med-QUEST Administration
820 Mililani Street, Suite 606
Honolulu, HI 96813
(808) 586-5391 phone
(808) 586-5389 fax

The state's hospital association can be contacted at:

Healthcare Association of Hawaii
932 Ward Avenue, Suite 430
Honolulu, HI 96814-2126
(808) 521-8961 phone
(808) 599-2879 fax

The state's insurance commissioner can be contacted at:

Acting State Insurance Commissioner
Hiram Tanaka
Insurance Division/Department of Commerce and Consumer Affairs
State of Hawaii
P.O. Box 3614
Honolulu, HI 96811-3614
(808) 586-2790 phone
(808) 586-2806 fax

Contact for health insurance information:
Shelley Santo
(808) 586-2809 phone

Contact for annual statement information:
Gale Yokomura
(808) 586-2804 phone

Please note: Before data are requested from any source, it is advisable to telephone the source to confirm that the data sought are available in the time period desired. In addition, the cost and exact procedure for obtaining data are most easily explained in a telephone conversation.

Idaho

State facility data are listed by hospital in the annual *Hospital Utilization Report.* In addition, specific requests for data taken from hospitals' annual reports will be honored. The general format for routine requests is paper; complex data requests are handled on a case-by-case basis, and can be on either paper or disk. Nursing home data (excluding ICF/MR) are also collected.

Requests for data should be directed to:

Chris Johnson, Health Policy Analyst
Center for Vital Statistics and Health Policy
450 West State Street, 1st Floor
P.O. Box 83720
Boise, ID 83720-0036
(208) 334-6571 phone
(208) 334-0685 fax

Medicare cost reports can be requested from:

Government Programs Division
Blue Cross and Blue Shield of Oregon
P.O. Box 8110
Portland, OR 97207-8110
(503) 721-7007 phone
(503) 228-3304 fax

The state's hospital association can be contacted at:

Idaho Hospital Association
P.O. Box 1278
Boise, ID 83701-1278
(208) 338-5100 phone
(208) 338-7800 fax

The state's insurance commissioner can be contacted at:

Acting State Insurance Commissioner
James M. Alcorn
Department of Insurance
State of Idaho
P.O. Box 83720
Boise, ID 83720-0043
(208) 334-4250 phone
(208) 334-4398 fax

Contact for health insurance information:
Joan Krosch
(208) 334-4250 phone

Contact for annual statement information:
Cyndi Sikorski
(208) 334-4250 phone

Please note: Before data are requested from any source, it is advisable to telephone the source to confirm that the data sought are available in the time period desired. In addition, the cost and exact procedure for obtaining data are most easily explained in a telephone conversation.

Illinois

The Facilities Planning Board inventories general hospitals by health service area and publishes a complete inventory list. Select clinical service discharges are listed by hospital. Separate volumes address general acute care and long-term care facilities.

Requests for patient-specific data on charges by ICD-9 code should be directed to:

Illinois Health Care Cost Containment Council
4500 South 6th Street Road, Suite 215
Springfield, IL 62703-5118
(217) 786-7001 phone

Requests for copies of the inventories or for specific data should be directed to:

Health Facilities Planning Board
525 West Jefferson Street, 2nd Floor
Springfield, IL 62761
(217) 782-3516 phone
(217) 785-4308 fax

Illinois participates in an Agency for Health Care Policy and Research project called the Healthcare Cost and Utilization Project (HCUP-3). HCUP-3 has created the State Inpatient Database, which provides comparable inpatient data for 12 states: Arizona, California, Colorado, Florida, Illinois, Iowa, Massachusetts, New Jersey, New York, Pennsylvania, Washington, and Wisconsin. Each state has established policies and procedures for gaining access to state data. Requests related to the Illinois HCUP-3 State Inpatient Database should be directed to:

John Noak
Illinois Health Care Cost Containment Council
4500 South 6th Street Road, Suite 215
Springfield, IL 62703-5118
(217) 786-7001 phone
(217) 786-7179 fax

If information is needed regarding the HCUP-3 project in general, please contact the Agency for Health Care Policy and Research, Division of Provider Studies, Center for Intramural Research, (301) 594-1410 (phone), (301) 594-2314 (fax), hcupSID@cghsir.ahcpr.gov (via Internet).

Medicare cost reports can be requested from:

Health Care Service Corporation
Attention: Robert Frederick, Provider and Audit Department
 (Blue Cross and Blue Shield–Illinois Medicare)
P.O. Box 2462
Chicago, IL 60690
(312) 938-6300 phone
(312) 540-0173 fax

The state's hospital association can be contacted at:

Illinois Hospital and Health Systems Association
1151 East Warrenville Road
P.O. Box 3015
Naperville, IL 60566
(708) 505-7777 phone
(708) 505-9457 fax

The state's insurance commissioner can be contacted at:

State Insurance Commissioner
James W. Schacht
Department of Insurance
State of Illinois
320 West Washington Street, 4th Floor
Springfield, IL 62767
(217) 782-4515 phone
(217) 782-5020 fax

Contact for health insurance information:
Ron Kotowski
(217) 782-4254 phone

Contact for annual statement information:
James Fassero
(217) 782-1759 phone

Please note: Before data are requested from any source, it is advisable to telephone the source to confirm that the data sought are available in the time period desired. In addition, the cost and exact procedure for obtaining data are most easily explained in a telephone conversation.

Indiana

Utilization and financial statistics are collected and disseminated by the state's Health Planning Division. All collected data are available on paper. Admission and discharge data as well as surgery data are available in electronic format and have detail at the ICD-9 level. As of July 1995, Indiana will be a UB-92 state.

Requests for data should be directed to:

Tom Reed
Director, Health Planning Division
Indiana State Board of Health
Room 334W
1330 West Michigan Street, P.O. Box 1964
Indianapolis, IN 46206-1964
(317) 383-6541 phone
(317) 383-6489 fax

The state's Medicare intermediary is:

Anthem Health Systems
Blue Cross and Blue Shield of Indiana
5451 West Lakeview Parkway South Drive
Indianapolis, IN 46268
(800) 345-4344 phone
(317) 290-5695 fax

The state's hospital association can be contacted at:

Indiana Hospital Association
One American Square
P.O. Box 82063
Indianapolis, IN 46282
(317) 633-4870 phone
(317) 633-4875 fax

Publicly available data are distributed by the Indiana State Department of Health. The state's insurance commissioner can be contacted at:

State Insurance Commissioner
Donna Bennett
Department of Insurance
311 West Washington Street, Suite 300
Indianapolis, IN 46204-2787
(317) 232-2385 phone
(317) 232-5251 fax

Contact for health insurance information:
Margaret McAllan
(317) 232-2418 phone

Contact for annual statement information:
Eric Sabotin
(317) 232-0689 phone

Please note: Before data are requested from any source, it is advisable to telephone the source to confirm that the data sought are available in the time period desired. In addition, the cost and exact procedure for obtaining data are most easily explained in a telephone conversation.

Iowa

The Iowa Office of Health Planning administers the annual AHA hospital survey. In addition, the Iowa Data Commission collects claims-based data from third-party payers on inpatient, outpatient, and physician/surgical services. Standard reports are available, and special requests will be handled on a case-by-case basis. Data tapes are updated yearly.

Iowa participates in an Agency for Health Care Policy and Research project called the Healthcare Cost and Utilization Project (HCUP-3). HCUP-3 has created the State Inpatient Database, which provides comparable inpatient data for 12 states: Arizona, California, Colorado, Florida, Illinois, Iowa, Massachusetts, New Jersey, New York, Pennsylvania, Washington, and Wisconsin. Each state has established policies and procedures for gaining access to state data. Requests related to the Iowa HCUP-3 State Inpatient Database should be directed to:

Jeanean Hood
Iowa Hospital Association
100 East Grand Avenue, Suite 100
Des Moines, IA 50309
(515) 288-1955 phone
(515) 283-9366 fax

If information is needed regarding the HCUP-3 project in general, please contact the Agency for Health Care Policy and Research, Division of Provider Studies, Center for Intramural Research, (301) 594-1410 (phone), (301) 594-2314 (fax), hcupSID@cghsir.ahcpr.gov (via Internet).

Requests for state-level data should be directed to:

Jeff Petrie
Vice-President
Health Management Information Center
601 Locust, Suite 330
Des Moines, IA 50310
(515) 244-1211 phone
(515) 288-9143 fax

Other requests for data should be directed to:

Pierce Wilson, Management Analyst
Office of Health Planning
Department of Public Health
Lucas State Office Building
321 East 12th Street
Des Moines, IA 50319-0075
(515) 281-4346 phone
(515) 281-4958 fax

Medicare cost reports can be requested from:

Blue Cross of Western Iowa and South Dakota
636 Grand Avenue, Station 28
Des Moines, IA 50309-2565
(515) 245-7538 phone
(515) 245-3965 fax

The state's hospital association can be contacted at:

Steve Brenton, President
Iowa Hospital Association
100 East Grand Avenue, Suite 100
Des Moines, IA 50309
(515) 288-1955 phone
(515) 283-9366 fax

Data contact person:

Diana Fuller
Iowa Hospital Association
100 East Grand Avenue, Suite 100
Des Moines, IA 50322
(515) 283-9322 phone
(515) 283-9366 fax

Data are available by DRG or ICD-9 code on paper or diskette. The charge varies according to the data requested.

The state's insurance commissioner can be contacted at:

State Insurance Commissioner
Therese Vaughan
Division of Insurance
State of Iowa
Lucas State Office Building, 6th Floor
Des Moines, IA 50319
(515) 281-5705 phone
(515) 281-3059 fax

Contact for health insurance information:
Roger Strauss
(515) 281-8245 phone

Contact for annual statement information:
Robert Howe
(515) 281-4450 phone

Please note: Before data are requested from any source, it is advisable to telephone the source to confirm that the data sought are available in the time period desired. In addition, the cost and exact procedure for obtaining data are most easily explained in a telephone conversation.

Kansas

Kansas is currently developing a health care database. Statewide hospital admissions data (by unit) and limited financial data are now collected.

Requests for data should be directed to:

Elizabeth W. Saadi
Director, Office of Health Care Information
Center for Health and Environmental Statistics
Kansas Department of Health and Environment
109 SW 9th Street
Mills Building, Suite 400A
Topeka, KS 66612-2219
(913) 296-5639 phone
(913) 296-7025 fax
uskanjdv@ibmmail.com e-mail

Medicare cost reports can be requested from:

Blue Cross and Blue Shield of Kansas, Inc.
1133 SW Topeka Boulevard
Topeka, KS 66629
(913) 291-7000 phone
(913) 291-8465 fax

The state's hospital association can be contacted at:

Kansas Hospital Association
1263 Topeka Avenue
P.O. Box 2308
Topeka, KS 66601
(913) 233-7436 phone
(913) 233-6955 fax

Data collected are released only to Kansas member hospitals or through the *Profiles of Kansas Hospitals* published by the association annually.

The state's insurance commissioner can be contacted at:

State Insurance Commissioner
Ron Todd
Department of Insurance
State of Kansas
420 SW 9th Street
Topeka, KS 66612-1678
(913) 296-3071 phone
(913) 296-2283 fax

Contact for health insurance information:
Richard G. Huncker
(913) 296-7850 phone

Contact for annual statement information:
Richard G. Huncker
(913) 296-7850 phone

Please note: Before data are requested from any source, it is advisable to telephone the source to confirm that the data sought are available in the time period desired. In addition, the cost and exact procedure for obtaining data are most easily explained in a telephone conversation.

Kentucky

DRG-level or ICD-9-level detail is not available for Kentucky data. Data are available on paper only.

Requests for state-level data should be directed to:

Michael J. Hammons
Kentucky Health Policy Board
3572 Iron Works Pike
Lexington, KY 40511
(606) 281-1213 phone
(606) 281-1511 fax

Other requests for data should be directed to:

Department of Health Services
Health Services Building
Health Data Branch
275 East Main Street, 1 East
Frankfort, KY 40621
(502) 564-2757 phone
(502) 564-6533 fax

Medicare cost reports can be requested from:

Blue Cross and Blue Shield of Kentucky, Inc.
9901 Linn Station Road
Louisville, KY 40223
(502) 423-2498 phone
(502) 329-8544 fax

The state's hospital association can be contacted at:

Kentucky Hospital Association
1302 Clear Spring Trace
P.O. Box 24163
Louisville, KY 40224
(502) 426-6220 phone
(502) 426-6226 fax

The state's insurance commissioner can be contacted at:

State Insurance Commissioner
Don W. Stephens
Department of Insurance
Commonwealth of Kentucky
P.O. Box 517
215 West Main Street
Frankfort, KY 40602
(502) 564-6027 phone
(502) 564-6090 fax

Contact for health insurance information:
Mike Johnston
(502) 564-6088 phone

Contact for annual statement information:
Windell Clark
(502) 564-6082 phone

Please note: Before data are requested from any source, it is advisable to telephone the source to confirm that the data sought are available in the time period desired. In addition, the cost and exact procedure for obtaining data are most easily explained in a telephone conversation.

Louisiana

Louisiana does not collect financial or utilization data. The annual AHA survey is administered by the Louisiana Hospital Association, which releases information only to contributing hospitals.

Medicare cost reports can be requested from:

Arkansas Blue Cross and Blue Shield
Medicare Services
P.O. Box 98501
Baton Rouge, LA 70884-9501
(504) 529-1494 phone
(504) 231-2124 fax

The state's hospital association can be contacted at:

Louisiana Hospital Association
P.O. Box 80720
Baton Rouge, LA 70898-0720
(504) 928-0026 phone
(504) 923-1004 fax

The state's insurance commissioner can be contacted at:

State Insurance Commissioner
James H. Brown
Department of Insurance
State of Louisiana
P.O. Box 94214
Baton Rouge, LA 70804-9214
(504) 342-5900 phone
(504) 342-3078 fax

Contact for health insurance information:
Pam Williams
(504) 342-1259 phone

Contact for annual statement information:
Cheryl Turrentine
(504) 342-1209 phone

Please note: Before data are requested from any source, it is advisable to telephone the source to confirm that the data sought are available in the time period desired. In addition, the cost and exact procedure for obtaining data are most easily explained in a telephone conversation.

Maine

Inpatient data are available by DRG or ICD-9 code on paper, tape, or diskette. Extensive outpatient utilization data are also collected. The charge varies according to the data requested.

Requests for data should be directed to:

Director, Division of Research and Data Management
Maine Health Care Finance Commission
State House Station #102
Augusta, ME 04333
(207) 287-3006 phone
(207) 287-6327 fax

Medicare cost reports can be requested from:

Associated Hospital Service of Maine
Maine Blue Cross and Blue Shield
2 Gannett Drive
South Portland, ME 04106-6911
(207) 822-8181 phone
(207) 822-7375 fax

The state's hospital association can be contacted at:

Maine Hospital Association
150 Capitol Street
Augusta, ME 04330
(207) 622-4794 phone
(207) 622-3073 fax

The state's insurance commissioner can be contacted at:

State Insurance Commissioner
Brian K. Atchinson
Department of Professional and Financial Regulation
Bureau of Insurance, State of Maine
State House Station #34
Augusta, ME 04333-0034
(207) 582-8707 phone
(207) 582-8716 fax

Contact for health insurance information:
Dave Stetson
(207) 582-8707 phone

Contact for annual statement information:
Lisa Nelson
(207) 582-8707 phone

Please note: Before data are requested from any source, it is advisable to telephone the source to confirm that the data sought are available in the time period desired. In addition, the cost and exact procedure for obtaining data are most easily explained in a telephone conversation.

Maryland

Data are available by DRG or ICD-9 code on paper or diskette. All financial data are from annual audited financial statements for Maryland hospitals. The charge varies according to the data requested.

Requests for hospital-level data should be directed to:

Theressa Lee
Administrator
Maryland Health Services Cost Review Council
4201 Patterson Avenue, 2nd Floor
Baltimore, MD 21215
(410) 764-2577 phone
(410) 764-5987 fax

Other requests for data should be directed to:

Andrea Albrecht
Director of Information Services
Maryland Hospital Association
1301 York Road, Suite 800
Lutherville, MD 21093
(410) 321-6200 phone
(410) 321-6268 fax

Medicare cost reports can be requested from:

Blue Cross and Blue Shield of Maryland, Inc.
10455 Mill Run Circle
Owings Mills, MD 21117
(410) 581-3000 phone
(410) 998-4502 fax

The state's hospital association can be contacted at:

Maryland Hospital Association
1301 York Road, Suite 800
Lutherville, MD 21093-6087
(410) 321-6200 phone
(410) 321-6268 fax

The state's insurance commissioner can be contacted at:

State Insurance Commissioner
Dwight K. Bartlett, III
Maryland Insurance Administration
501 St. Paul Place, 7th Floor-South
Baltimore, MD 21202-2272
(410) 333-2521 phone
(410) 333-6650 fax

Contact for health insurance information:
Randi Reichel
(410) 333-4968 phone

Contact for annual statement information:
William Lashley
(410) 333-6196 phone

Please note: Before data are requested from any source, it is advisable to telephone the source to confirm that the data sought are available in the time period desired. In addition, the cost and exact procedure for obtaining data are most easily explained in a telephone conversation.

Massachusetts

Massachusetts collects UB92-level data on all hospital discharges in the state. The data are available to the public in electronic format after a specific request is made. Diagnosis and procedure-level detail is available as well as diagnosis-related group (DRG) classification. The cost per request varies according to the level of complexity of the request.

In addition, Massachusetts participates in an Agency for Health Care Policy and Research project called the Healthcare Cost and Utilization Project (HCUP-3). HCUP-3 has created the State Inpatient Database, which provides comparable inpatient data for 12 states: Arizona, California, Colorado, Florida, Illinois, Iowa, Massachusetts, New Jersey, New York, Pennsylvania, Washington, and Wisconsin. Each state has established policies and procedures for gaining access to state data. Requests related to the Massachusetts HCUP-3 State Inpatient Database, as well as most other requests for data, should be directed to:

David Stachelski
Massachusetts Rate Setting Commission
2 Boylston Street
Boston, MA 02116
(617) 451-5330 phone
(617) 451-1878 fax

If information is needed regarding the HCUP-3 project in general, please contact the Agency for Health Care Policy and Research, Division of Provider Studies, Center for Intramural Research, (301) 594-1410 (phone), (301) 594-2314 (fax), hcupSID@cghsir.ahcpr.gov (via Internet).

Requests for hospital-level data should be directed to:

Gene Delahanty
Data Analyst
Hospital Bureau
Massachusetts Rate Setting Commission
2 Boylston Street
Boston, MA 02116
(617) 451-5330 phone
(617) 451-1878 fax

Medicare cost reports can be requested from:

Medicare/Blue Shield of Massachusetts, Inc.
22 Richards Road
Plymouth, MA 02363
(508) 747-3080 phone
(508) 830-4900 fax

The state's hospital association can be contacted at:

Massachusetts Hospital Association
Five New England Executive Park
Burlington, MA 01803
(617) 272-8000 phone
(617) 272-0466 fax

The state's insurance commissioner can be contacted at:

State Insurance Commissioner
Linda Ruthardt
Division of Insurance
Commonwealth of Massachusetts
470 Atlantic Avenue, 6th Floor
Boston, MA 02210-2223
(617) 521-7794 phone
(617) 521-7770 fax

Contact for health insurance information:
Cameron McIntosh, Acting Director
(617) 521-7349 phone

Contact for annual statement information:
Peter Arens
(617) 521-7392 phone

Please note: Before data are requested from any source, it is advisable to telephone the source to confirm that the data sought are available in the time period desired. In addition, the cost and exact procedure for obtaining data are most easily explained in a telephone conversation.

Michigan

Data are available by ICD-9 code on paper, tape, or diskette. The charge varies according to the data requested.

Requests for data should be directed to:

Stanley I. Nash,
Chief Survey and Statistical Studies Section
Office of State Registrar and Center for Health Statistics
3423 North Logan/Martin Luther King, Jr. Boulevard
P.O. Box 30195
Lansing, MI 48909
(517) 335-8587 phone
(517) 335-8711 fax

Medicare cost reports can be requested from:

Blue Cross and Blue Shield of Michigan
P.O. Box 2500
Detroit, MI 48226
(313) 225-8000 phone
(313) 225-6239 fax

The state's hospital association can be contacted at:

Michigan Health & Hospital Association
6215 West St. Joseph Highway
Lansing, MI 48917
(517) 323-3443 phone
(517) 323-0946 fax

The Michigan Hospital Association assists the AHA with the Annual Survey of Hospitals data collection in Michigan. The data are reported in various publications targeted to hospitals and the general public. Hospital-specific data are not reported unless they appear in public resources in hospital-specific format. Other requests for hospital-specific data are reviewed by the Michigan Hospital Association.

Data are available on paper, magnetic tape, and diskette. The charge varies according to the data requested.

The state's insurance commissioner can be contacted at:

State Insurance Commissioner
David Dykhouse
Insurance Bureau/Department of Commerce
State of Michigan
P.O. Box 30220
Lansing, MI 48909-7720
(517) 373-9273 phone
(517) 335-4978 fax

Contact for health insurance information:
Frances Wallace
(517) 335-2057 phone

Contact for annual statement information:
Mary Lewis
(517) 335-4501 phone

Please note: Before data are requested from any source, it is advisable to telephone the source to confirm that the data sought are available in the time period desired. In addition, the cost and exact procedure for obtaining data are most easily explained in a telephone conversation.

Minnesota

The Facility and Provider Compliance Division collects extensive utilization data for the Annual Statistical Report to the Commission of Health. Data extracted from the report are charged at $18.00 per hour and $.05 per sheet. Nursing home data became available as of the last quarter of 1994.

Requests for hospital-level data should be directed to:

Jim Golden
Manager, Data Analysis Program
Health Care Delivery Policy Division
Minnesota Department of Health
121 East 7th Place, Suite 400
P.O. Box 64975
St. Paul, MN 55164-0975
(612) 282-5640 phone
(612) 282-5628 fax

Walter Suarez
Director of Operations
Minnesota Health Data Institute
910 Piper Jaffray Tower
444 Cedar Street
St. Paul, MN 55101
(612) 228-4372 phone
(612) 222-4209 fax

Other requests for data should be directed to:

Jeanie Schaffer, Health Program Aide
Surveying and Licensing Section
Facility and Provider Compliance Division
393 North Dunlap Street, Box 64900
St. Paul, MN 55164-0900
(612) 643-2100 phone
(612) 643-3534 fax

Medicare cost reports can be requested from:

Blue Cross and Blue Shield of Minnesota
P.O. Box 64560
St. Paul, MN 55164
(612) 456-8454 phone
(612) 683-2162 fax

The state's hospital association can be contacted at:

Minnesota Hospital Association
2221 University Avenue S.E., Suite 425
Minneapolis, MN 55414-3085
(612) 331-5571 phone
(612) 331-1001 fax

Data contact person:

Mitch Davis
Manager, HIRM
Suite 425
2221 University Avenue S.E.
Minneapolis, MN 55414-3085

Data are available on paper or diskette. The charge varies according to the data requested.

The state's insurance commissioner can be contacted at:

State Insurance Commissioner
James E. Ulland
Department of Commerce
State of Minnesota
133 East 7th Street
St. Paul, MN 55101
(612) 296-6848 phone
(612) 296-4328 fax

Contact for health insurance information:
John Gross
(612) 296-6929 phone

Contact for annual statement information:
Kathleen Orme
(612) 297-7161

Please note: Before data are requested from any source, it is advisable to telephone the source to confirm that the data sought are available in the time period desired. In addition, the cost and exact procedure for obtaining data are most easily explained in a telephone conversation.

Mississippi

The State Department of Health collects hospital utilization data. They do not use ICD-9 codes or DRGs, nor do they collect financial data.
    Requests for data should be directed to:

Gay Simpson
Mississippi State Department of Health
P.O. Box 1700
Jackson, MS 39215-1700
(601) 960-7978 phone

        Medicare cost reports can be requested from:

Blue Cross and Blue Shield of Mississippi
P.O. Box 23035
Jackson, MS 39225-3035
(601) 932-3704 phone
(601) 932-9233 fax

        The state's hospital association can be contacted at:

Mississippi Hospital Association
P.O. Box 16444
Jackson, MS 39236-6444
(601) 982-3251 phone
(601) 366-3962 fax

        The state's insurance commissioner can be contacted at:

State Insurance Commissioner
George Dale
Department of Insurance
State of Mississippi
P.O. Box 79
Jackson, MS 39205
(601) 359-3569 phone
(601) 359-2474 fax

Contact for health insurance information:
Cathy Vernon
(601) 359-2130 phone

Contact for annual statement information:
Jimmy Blissett
(601) 359-2139 phone

Please note: Before data are requested from any source, it is advisable to telephone the source to confirm that the data sought are available in the time period desired. In addition, the cost and exact procedure for obtaining data are most easily explained in a telephone conversation.

Missouri

Patient-level charge data are available for hospitals and ambulatory surgical centers. Some limited utilization data are available for nursing home/residential care facilities. For nonfinancial hospital utilization data, contact M. J. Mosley at (314) 751-6279. For financial data, contact Barbara Hoskins or Norma Helmig. Contact Barbara Hoskins for patient-level data.

Requests for data should be directed to:

Barbara Hoskins
Chief, Bureau of Health Resources Statistics
State of Missouri
Department of Health/Division of Health Resources
P.O. Box 570
Jefferson City, MO 65102
(314) 751-6279 phone
(314) 751-6010 fax

Medicare cost reports can be requested from:

Eddy Price
Tri-Span
3545 Lakeland Drive
Jackson, MS 39208-9799
(601) 932-7777 ext. 4564 phone
(601) 939-1610 fax

The state's hospital association can be contacted at:

Missouri Hospital Association
4712 Country Club Drive
P.O. Box 60
Jefferson City, MO 65102
(314) 893-3700 phone
(314) 893-2809 fax

The state's insurance commissioner can be contacted at:

State Insurance Commissioner
Jay Angoff
Department of Insurance
State of Missouri
P.O. Box 690
Jefferson City, MO 65102
(314) 751-4126 phone
(314) 526-6075 fax

Contact for health insurance information:
James Casey
(314) 751-4363 phone

Contact for annual statement information:
Steve Divine
(314) 751-3497 phone

Please note: Before data are requested from any source, it is advisable to telephone the source to confirm that the data sought are available in the time period desired. In addition, the cost and exact procedure for obtaining data are most easily explained in a telephone conversation.

Montana

No utilization or financial data are available.
    Medicare cost reports can be requested from:

Blue Cross and Blue Shield of Montana
P.O. Box 4309
Helena, MT 59604
(406) 444-8200 phone
(406) 447-3454 fax

    The state's hospital association can be contacted at:

Montana Hospital Association
1720 9th Avenue
P.O. Box 5119
Helena, MT 59604
(406) 442-1911 phone
(406) 443-3894 fax

    The state's insurance commissioner can be contacted at:

State Insurance Commissioner
Mark O'Keefe
Department of Insurance
State of Montana
126 North Sanders/Mitchell Building, Room 270
Helena, MT 59620
(406) 444-2040 phone
(406) 444-3497 fax

Contact for health insurance information:
Louise Ford
(406) 444-2040 phone

Contact for annual statement information:
James Borchardt
(406) 444-2040 phone

Please note: Before data are requested from any source, it is advisable to telephone
the source to confirm that the data sought are available in the time period desired.
In addition, the cost and exact procedure for obtaining data are most easily
explained in a telephone conversation.

Nebraska

Data are available on paper or floppy disk. Paper data are charged at $0.75 for the first page and $0.15 per page thereafter, and electronic data charges depend on the request. Nursing home utilization data are also available.

Requests for data should be directed to:

Kathy Kelly, Data Coordinator
Health Policy and Planning
Nebraska Department of Health
301 Centennial Mall, Box 95007
Lincoln, NE 68509-5007
(402) 471-2337 phone
(402) 471-0180 fax

Medicare cost reports can be requested from:

Arlene Ropers, Fiscal Project Analyst
Nebraska Department of Social Services
301 Centennial Mall South, 5th Floor
P.O. Box 95026
Lincoln, NE 68509-5026
(402) 471-9159 phone
(402) 471-9455 fax

The state's hospital association can be contacted at:

Nebraska Association of Hospitals and Health Systems
1640 L Street, Suite D
Lincoln, NE 68508-2509
(402) 476-0141 phone
(402) 475-4091 fax

The state's insurance commissioner can be contacted at:

State Insurance Commissioner
Robert G. Lange
Department of Insurance
State of Nebraska
941 'O' Street, Suite 400
Lincoln, NE 68508
(402) 471-2201 phone
(402) 471-4610 fax

Contact for health insurance information:
Ronald Elmshauser
(402) 471-4742 phone
(402) 471-6559 fax

Contact for annual statement information:
David Krumm
(402) 471-4641 phone

Please note: Before data are requested from any source, it is advisable to telephone the source to confirm that the data sought are available in the time period desired. In addition, the cost and exact procedure for obtaining data are most easily explained in a telephone conversation.

Nevada

The Nevada State Department of Human Resources collects and publishes hospital discharge data. Inpatient data are available by DRG and ICD-9 code on paper, tape, or floppy disk. The charge varies according to the data requested. Utilization data are also available for ambulatory surgery centers, skilled nursing facilities, and hospices.

Requests for data should be directed to:

Nevada Department of Human Resources
Health Care Financial Analysis Unit
505 East King Street, Room 604
Carson City, NV 89710
(702) 687-4176 phone
(702) 687-4733 fax

Medicare cost reports can be requested from:

Aetna Life and Casualty
Part A Medicare
P.O. Box 808019
Petaluma, CA 94975-8019
(800) 523-5051 phone
(707) 664-0365 phone

The state's hospital association can be contacted at:

Nevada Hospital Association
4600 Kietzke Lane, Suite A-108
Reno, NV 89502
(702) 827-0184 phone
(702) 827-0190 fax

The state's insurance commissioner can be contacted at:

State Insurance Commissioner
Teresa P. Froncek Rankin
Division of Insurance
Capitol Complex/State of Nevada
1665 Hot Spring Road, Suite 152
Carson City, NV 89710
(702) 687-4270 phone
(702) 687-3937 fax

Contact for health insurance information:
Sharen Weaver (Carson City)
(702) 687-7661 phone

Contact for annual statement information:
David J. Carbon
(702) 687-7684 phone

Please note: Before data are requested from any source, it is advisable to telephone the source to confirm that the data sought are available in the time period desired. In addition, the cost and exact procedure for obtaining data are most easily explained in a telephone conversation.

New Hampshire

Hospital inpatient and financial data are collected and disseminated by the Division of Public Health Services. Data are available by DRG and ICD-9 code and can be obtained on paper, tape, or disk.

Requests for data should be directed to:

Kenneth Roos
Health Data Service Unit
New Hampshire Division of Public Health Services
6 Hazen Drive
Concord, NH 03301
(603) 271-4671 phone
(603) 271-3745 fax

Medicare cost reports can be requested from:

New Hampshire Division of Human Services
6 Hazen Drive
Concord, NH 03301
(603) 271-4326 phone
(603) 271-4727 fax
or
New Hampshire–Vermont Health Service
3000 Goffs Falls Road
Manchester, NH 03111-0001
(603) 695-7000 phone
(603) 695-7095 fax

The state's hospital association can be contacted at:

Kathy Bizarro, Vice-President, Data Services
New Hampshire Hospital Association
125 Airport Road
Concord, NH 03301-5388
(603) 225-0900 phone
(603) 225-4346 fax

The state's insurance commissioner can be contacted at:

State Insurance Commissioner
Sylvio L. Dupuis
Department of Insurance
State of New Hampshire
169 Manchester Street
Concord, NH 03301-5151
(603) 271-2261 phone
(603) 271-1406 fax

Contact for health insurance information:
Robert C. Warren, Jr.
(603) 271-2261 phone

Contact for annual statement information:
Thomas Burke
(603) 271-2261 phone

Please note: Before data are requested from any source, it is advisable to telephone the source to confirm that the data sought are available in the time period desired. In addition, the cost and exact procedure for obtaining data are most easily explained in a telephone conversation.

New Jersey

The State Department of Health collects hospital utilization data. Data are also collected on psychiatric, children's rehabilitation, and long-term care facilities, as well as home health agencies. No financial data are collected. Data are not available by DRG or ICD-9 code. Paper is the only format available.

New Jersey participates in an Agency for Health Care Policy and Research project called the Healthcare Cost and Utilization Project (HCUP-3). HCUP-3 has created the State Inpatient Database, which provides comparable inpatient data for 12 states: Arizona, California, Colorado, Florida, Illinois, Iowa, Massachusetts, New Jersey, New York, Pennsylvania, Washington, and Wisconsin. Each state has established policies and procedures for gaining access to state data. Requests related to the New Jersey HCUP-3 State Inpatient Database should be directed to:

Vince Yarmlak
New Jersey State Department of Health
CN-360, Room 601
Trenton, NJ 08625-0360
(609) 984-7931 phone
(609) 292-3780 fax

If information is needed regarding the HCUP-3 project in general, please contact the Agency for Health Care Policy and Research, Division of Provider Studies, Center for Intramural Research, (301) 594-1410 (phone), (301) 594-2314 (fax), hcupSID@cghsir.ahcpr.gov (via Internet).

Requests for hospital-level data should be directed to:

Anne Davis
Office of Health Policy and Research
New Jersey State Department of Health
CN 360, Room 800
Trenton, NJ 08625-0360
(609) 292-7837 phone
(609) 292-0085 fax

Other requests for data should be directed to:

Ralph White, Research Scientist
New Jersey State Department of Health
Center for Health Statistics
CN-360, Room 405
Trenton, NJ 08625-0360
(609) 292-4055 phone
(609) 984-7633 fax

Medicare cost reports can be requested from:

Blue Cross and Blue Shield of New Jersey, Inc.
33 Washington Street—MS 04Y
Newark, NJ 07103
(201) 456-3020 phone
(201) 456-2899 fax

The state's hospital association can be contacted at:

New Jersey Hospital Association
Center for Health Affairs
746–760 Alexander Road, CN-1
Princeton, NJ 08543-0001
(609) 275-4000 phone
(609) 275-4100 fax

The state's insurance commissioner can be contacted at:

State Insurance Commissioner
Drew Karpinski
Department of Insurance
State of New Jersey
20 West State Street, CN 325
Trenton, NJ 08625
(609) 292-5363 phone
(609) 292-0896 fax

Contact for health insurance information:
Asutosh Chakrabarti
(609) 633-0523 phone

Contact for annual statement information:
Joann Jones
(609) 292-5468 phone

Please note: Before data are requested from any source, it is advisable to telephone the source to confirm that the data sought are available in the time period desired. In addition, the cost and exact procedure for obtaining data are most easily explained in a telephone conversation.

New Mexico

The New Mexico Health Policy Commission collects inpatient discharge data from all nonfederal, licensed general, and specialty hospitals in New Mexico. Data are primarily those available on a UB-92 form. Aggregate data by ICD-9 code will be provided in groups large enough to protect provider identities. No financial data will be collected. All requests for data need to identify specific codes or code ranges. The charge varies according to the data requested.

Requests for data should be directed to:

Ron Dirks
Health Information System Office
New Mexico Health Policy Commission
410 Don Gaspar
Santa Fe, NM 87501
(505) 827-4488 phone
(505) 827-4481 fax

Medicare cost reports can be requested from:

Blue Cross and Blue Shield of New Mexico
P.O. Box 27630
Albuquerque, NM 87125-7630
(505) 292-2600 phone
(505) 291-3541 fax

The state's hospital association can be contacted at:

New Mexico Hospitals and Health Systems Association
2121 Osuna Road NE
Albuquerque, NM 87113
(505) 343-0010 phone
(505) 343-0012 fax

Data contact person:

Terry Johnson, Health Data Analyst
New Mexico Hospitals and Health Systems Association
2121 Osuna Road NE
Albuquerque, NM 87113

Data are available on paper. The charge varies according to the data requested.

The state's insurance commissioner can be contacted at:

State Insurance Commissioner
Fabian Chavez
Department of Insurance
State of New Mexico
P.O. Drawer 1269
Santa Fe, NM 87504-1269
(505) 827-4601 phone
(505) 827-4734 fax

Contact for health insurance information:
Helen Hourdes
(505) 827-4545 phone

Contact for annual statement information:
James E. Scott
(505) 827-4655 phone

Please note: Before data are requested from any source, it is advisable to telephone the source to confirm that the data sought are available in the time period desired. In addition, the cost and exact procedure for obtaining data are most easily explained in a telephone conversation.

New York

The New York State Department of Health collects extensive hospital discharge and financial data. Most data are publicly accessible; however, every request for data is reviewed individually to determine eligibility for release under the state's Freedom of Information Act.

New York participates in an Agency for Health Care Policy and Research project called the Healthcare Cost and Utilization Project (HCUP-3). HCUP-3 has created the State Inpatient Database, which provides comparable inpatient data for 12 states: Arizona, California, Colorado, Florida, Illinois, Iowa, Massachusetts, New Jersey, New York, Pennsylvania, Washington, and Wisconsin. Each state has established policies and procedures for gaining access to state data. Requests related to the New York HCUP-3 State Inpatient Database, as well as requests for hospital-level data, should be directed to:

Gene Therriault
Bureau of Biometrics
New York State Department of Health
Room C144
Empire State Plaza
Albany, NY 12237-0044
(518) 474-3189 phone
(518) 486-1630 fax

If information is needed regarding the HCUP-3 project in general, please contact the Agency for Health Care Policy and Research, Division of Provider Studies, Center for Intramural Research, (301) 594-1410 (phone), (301) 594-2314 (fax), hcupSID@cghsir.ahcpr.gov (via Internet).

Requests for hospital-level data can also be directed to:

Michael Zdeb
New York State Department of Health
Empire State Tower
Room 890
Albany, NY 12237-0657
(518) 474-2079 phone
(518) 473-2015 fax

Other requests for data should be directed to:

Donald MacDonald, Records Access Officer
New York State Department of Health
Records Access Office
Corning Tower, Empire State Plaza
Albany, NY 12237
(518) 474-6936 phone
(518) 474-8163 fax

Medicare cost reports can be requested from:

Empire Blue Cross and Blue Shield Part A
P.O. Box 4846
Syracuse, NY 13221-4846
(315) 474-4159 phone
(315) 479-3054 fax

The state's hospital association can be contacted at:

Healthcare Association of New York State
74 North Pearl Street
Albany, NY 12207
(518) 431-7600 phone
(518) 431-7915 fax

The state's insurance commissioner can be contacted at:

State Insurance Commissioner
Salvatore R. Curiale
Department of Insurance
State of New York
160 West Broadway
New York, NY 10013
(212) 602-0429 phone
(212) 602-0437 fax

Contact for health insurance information:
Frederic Bodner
(518) 474-6272 phone

Contact for annual statement information:
James Hrbek
(518) 474-6615 phone

Please note: Before data are requested from any source, it is advisable to telephone the source to confirm that the data sought are available in the time period desired. In addition, the cost and exact procedure for obtaining data are most easily explained in a telephone conversation.

North Carolina

Data are sorted by DRG or ICD-9 code and are available on paper, magnetic tape, or diskette. The charge varies according to the data requested.

Requests for inpatient data should be directed to:

Executive Director
North Carolina Medical Database Commission
112 Cox Avenue, Suite 208
Raleigh, NC 27605
(919) 733-7141 phone
(919) 733-3682 fax

Requests for outpatient data should be directed to:

North Carolina Division of Facility Services
Attention: Medical Facilities Planners
Medical Facilities Planning Section
P.O. Box 29530
Raleigh, NC 27626-0503
(919) 733-4130 phone
(919) 733-2757 fax

Medicare cost reports can be requested from:

Blue Cross and Blue Shield of North Carolina
P.O. Box 2291
Durham, NC 27702
(919) 490-3360 phone
(919) 688-4973 fax

The state's hospital association can be contacted at:

North Carolina Hospital Association
P.O. Box 80428
Raleigh, NC 27623-0428
(919) 677-2400 phone
(919) 677-4200 fax

The state's insurance commissioner can be contacted at:

State Insurance Commissioner
Jim Long
Department of Insurance
State of North Carolina
P.O. Box 26387
Raleigh, NC 27611
(919) 733-7349 phone
(919) 733-6495 fax

Contact for health insurance information:
Wake Hamrick
(919) 733-5060 phone

Contact for annual statement information:
Terry Wade
(919) 733-5633 phone

Please note: Before data are requested from any source, it is advisable to telephone the source to confirm that the data sought are available in the time period desired. In addition, the cost and exact procedure for obtaining data are most easily explained in a telephone conversation.

North Dakota

North Dakota has detailed information on inpatient discharges available by DRG and ICD-9 code, on paper, tape, or floppy disk. A database covering one year of data may be purchased for $750.00. There is a charge of $25.00 per hour for custom report generation.

Requests for data should be directed to:

Gary Garland
North Dakota State Department of Health
600 East Boulevard Avenue
Bismarck, ND 58505-0200
(701) 328-2894 phone
(701) 328-4727 fax

Medicare cost reports can be requested from:

Attention: Pat Redlin
Provider Audit
Blue Cross of North Dakota
4510 13th Avenue SW
Fargo, ND 58121-0001
(701) 282-1216 phone
(701) 277-2449 fax

The state's hospital association can be contacted at:

North Dakota Hospital Association
1120 College Drive
P.O. Box 7340
Bismark, ND 58507-7340
(701) 224-9732 phone
(701) 224-9529 fax

The state's insurance commissioner can be contacted at:

State Insurance Commissioner
Glenn Pomeroy
Department of Insurance
State of North Dakota
600 East Boulevard Avenue
Bismarck, ND 58505-0320
(701) 328-2440 phone
(701) 328-4880 fax

Contact for health insurance information:
Vance Magnuson
(701) 328-4977 phone

Contact for annual statement information:
Leona Femling
(701) 328-2445 phone

Please note: Before data are requested from any source, it is advisable to telephone the source to confirm that the data sought are available in the time period desired. In addition, the cost and exact procedure for obtaining data are most easily explained in a telephone conversation.

Ohio

Inpatient admission/discharge data are available by DRG code on floppy disk. No financial data are available. A charge of $250.00 for statewide data or $35.00 by region is made.

Requests for data should be directed to:

Attention: Lorin Ranbom
Office of Health Policy and Analysis
Ohio Department of Health
246 North High Street
Columbus, OH 43266
(614) 466-5308 phone
(614) 644-8526 fax

Medicare cost reports can be requested from:

Diana Feldman-Smith, Manager
Community Mutual Insurance Company
801 A West 8th Street
P.O. Box 145482
Cincinnati, OH 45250-5482
(513) 852-4236 phone
(513) 852-4325 fax

Note: The Community Mutual Insurance Company does not handle claims assigned to Aetna.

The state's hospital association can be contacted at:

Ohio Hospital Association
155 East Broad Street
Columbus, OH 43215
(614) 221-7614 phone
(614) 221-4771 fax

The state's insurance commissioner can be contacted at:

State Insurance Commissioner
Harold T. Duryee
Department of Insurance
State of Ohio
2100 Stella Court
Columbus, OH 43215-1067
(614) 644-2658 phone
(614) 644-3743 fax

Contact for health insurance information:
Randy Ward
(614) 644-2644 phone

Contact for annual statement information:
William Rossbach
(614) 644-2647 phone

Please note: Before data are requested from any source, it is advisable to telephone the source to confirm that the data sought are available in the time period desired. In addition, the cost and exact procedure for obtaining data are most easily explained in a telephone conversation.

Oklahoma

Requests for data should be directed to:

Matthew K. Lucas
Director
Division of Health Care Information
Oklahoma Health Care Authority
4545 North Lincoln Boulevard, Suite 124
Oklahoma City, OK 73105
(405) 530-3439 phone
(405) 528-2786 fax

Medicare cost reports can be requested from:

Group Health Service of Oklahoma, Inc.
1215 South Boulder Avenue
Tulsa, OK 74119
(918) 560-3535 phone
(918) 560-7879 fax

The state's hospital association can be contacted at:

Oklahoma Hospital Association
4000 Lincoln Boulevard
Oklahoma City, OK 73105
(405) 427-9537 phone
(405) 424-4507 fax

The state's insurance commissioner can be contacted at:

State Insurance Commissioner
Catherine J. Weatherford
Department of Insurance
State of Oklahoma
P.O. Box 53408
Oklahoma City, OK 73152-3408
(405) 521-2828 phone
(405) 521-6635 fax

Contact for health insurance information:
Lynn Rambo-Jones
(405) 521-3541 phone

Contact for annual statement information:
Chris Perry
(405) 521-3966 phone

Please note: Before data are requested from any source, it is advisable to telephone the source to confirm that the data sought are available in the time period desired. In addition, the cost and exact procedure for obtaining data are most easily explained in a telephone conversation.

Oregon

The Oregon Department of Human Resources collects extensive hospital utilization and financial data. Inpatient data are available by DRG and ICD-9 code and are available on either paper or tape. All other information is available on paper or disk.

Requests for data should be directed to:

Ali Motidi, Research Analyst
State Office of Health Policy
Department of Human Resources
800 Northeast Oregon Street, Suite 640
Portland, OR 97232
(503) 731-4091 phone
(503) 731-4056 fax

Medicare cost reports can be requested from:

Blue Cross and Blue Shield of Oregon
100 Southwest Market Street
P.O. Box 1271
Portland, OR 97201
(503) 225-5336 phone
(503) 225-5232 fax

The state's hospital association can be contacted at:

Oregon Association of Hospitals and Health Systems
4000 Kruse Way Place
Building 2, Suite 100
Lake Oswego, OR 97035-2543
(503) 636-2204 phone
(503) 636-8310 fax

The Oregon Association of Hospitals and Health Systems collects both utilization and financial data. Call for availability.

The state's insurance commissioner can be contacted at:

State Insurance Commissioner
Kerry Barnett
Department of Consumer and Business Services
Director's Office
200 Labor and Industries Building
Salem, OR 97310
(503) 378-4120 phone
(503) 378-6444 fax

Contact for health insurance information:
Bill Sandhu
(503) 378-4481 ext. 630 phone

Contact for annual statement information:
Day Manion
(503) 378-4281 ext. 620 phone

Please note: Before data are requested from any source, it is advisable to telephone the source to confirm that the data sought are available in the time period desired. In addition, the cost and exact procedure for obtaining data are most easily explained in a telephone conversation.

Pennsylvania

The Department of Health publishes a directory of Pennsylvania hospitals biennially. Data for all hospitals licensed by the Department of Health are collected through an annual hospital questionnaire. A number of unpublished annual reports for fiscal years 1978–1992 containing data listed in appendixes A–C are available upon request, as is a directory of those reports. Data collected on the questionnaire but not in the reports are also available by special request. The charge for data varies according to the type of data and format.

Requests for a listing of reports available should be directed to:

Wendy Smith
Pennsylvania Department of Health
State Center for Health Statistics and Research
P.O. Box 90, Room 126
Harrisburg, PA 17108
(717) 783-2548 phone
(717) 772-3258 fax

Other information may be available and obtained by special request to the same office.

Pennsylvania participates in an Agency for Health Care Policy and Research project called the Healthcare Cost and Utilization Project (HCUP-3). HCUP-3 has created the State Inpatient Database, which provides comparable inpatient data for 12 states: Arizona, California, Colorado, Florida, Illinois, Iowa, Massachusetts, New Jersey, New York, Pennsylvania, Washington, and Wisconsin. Each state has established policies and procedures for gaining access to state data. Requests related to the Pennsylvania HCUP-3 State Inpatient Database, as well as other requests for state-level data, should be directed to:

Ernie Sessa
Pennsylvania Health Care Cost Containment Council
225 Market Street, Suite 400
Harrisburg, PA 17101
(717) 232-6787 phone
(717) 232-3821 fax

If information is needed regarding the HCUP-3 project in general, please contact the Agency for Health Care Policy and Research, Division of Provider Studies, Center for Intramural Research, (301) 594-1410 (phone), (301) 594-2314 (fax), hcupSID@cghsir.ahcpr.gov (via Internet).

Medicare cost reports can be requested from:

Veritus Inc.
Freedom of Information Office
Fifth Avenue Place
120 Fifth Avenue, Suite F8221
Pittsburgh, PA 15222-3099
(412) 928-3986 phone
(412) 928-3973 fax

Note: The counties of Bucks, Chester, Delaware, Montgomery, and Philadelphia are handled through the following office.

Independence Blue Cross
1901 Market Street
Philadelphia, PA 19103
(215) 241-2400 phone
(215) 241-3824 fax

The state's hospital association can be contacted at:

Hospital Association of Pennsylvania
4750 Lindle Road
P.O. Box 8600
Harrisburg, PA 17111-2428
(717) 564-9200 phone
(717) 561-5333 fax

The state's insurance commissioner can be contacted at:

State Insurance Commissioner
Cynthia M. Maleski
Department of Insurance
Commonwealth of Pennsylvania
1326 Strawberry Square, 13th Floor
Harrisburg, PA 17120
(717) 783-0442 phone
(717) 783-1059 fax

Contact for health insurance information:
Martha Bergsten
(717) 787-4192 phone

Contact for annual statement information:
Willard Smith
(717) 787-5890 phone

Please note: Before data are requested from any source, it is advisable to telephone the source to confirm that the data sought are available in the time period desired. In addition, the cost and exact procedure for obtaining data are most easily explained in a telephone conversation.

Rhode Island

Requests for data should be directed to:

Jay Buechner
Office of Health Statistics
3 Capitol Hill
Providence, RI 02908
(401) 277-2550 phone
(401) 277-6548 fax

Medicare cost reports can be requested from:

Blue Cross and Blue Shield of Rhode Island
444 Westminster Street
Providence, RI 02903
(401) 459-1400 phone
(401) 459-1598 fax

The state's hospital association can be contacted at:

Hospital Association of Rhode Island
880 Butler Drive, Suite One
Providence, RI 02906
(401) 453-8400 phone
(401) 453-8411 fax

The state's insurance commissioner can be contacted at:

State Insurance Commissioner
Alfonso Mastrostefano
Department of Insurance
Department of Business Regulation
State of Rhode Island
233 Richmond Street, Suite 233
Providence, RI 02903-4233
(401) 277-2223 phone
(401) 751-4887 fax

Contact for health insurance information:
G. Rollin Bartlett
(401) 277-2223 phone

Contact for annual statement information:
James Abraham
(401) 277-2223 phone

Please note: Before data are requested from any source, it is advisable to telephone the source to confirm that the data sought are available in the time period desired. In addition, the cost and exact procedure for obtaining data are most easily explained in a telephone conversation.

South Carolina

There are two primary sources of hospital data: an annual survey (similar to the AHA annual survey) and the Statewide Hospital Discharge Data System. Information from the annual survey is available to the public. Information from the Discharge Data System, which can be grouped by DRG or ICD-9 code, is subject to confidentiality restrictions, and requests for data are handled on a case-by-case basis. Data are available on paper, magnetic tape, or diskette, and the charge varies according to the data requested. For a list of standard data products from the Discharge Data System, contact the following address.

Requests for data should be directed to:

Beth Corley, Executive Manager, Health and Demographic Statistics
South Carolina Budget and Control Board
Office of Research and Statistical Services
1000 Assembly Street, Suite 425
Columbia, SC 29201-3117
(803) 734-3818 phone
(803) 734-3619 fax

Medicare cost reports can be requested from:

Bruce W. Hughes
Vice-President, Medicare Operations
Blue Cross and Blue Shield of South Carolina
P.O. Box 100190
Columbia, SC 29202
(803) 788-0222 ext. 1046 phone
(803) 788-8240 fax

The state's hospital association can be contacted at:

South Carolina Hospital Association
101 Medical Circle
P.O. Box 6009
West Columbia, SC 29171-6009
(803) 796-3080 phone
(803) 796-2938 fax

The state's insurance commissioner can be contacted at:

State Insurance Commissioner
John G. Richards
Department of Insurance
State of South Carolina
1612 Marion Street
Box 100105
Columbia, SC 29202
(803) 737-6160 phone
(803) 737-6205 fax

Contact for health insurance information:
C. Michael Jordan
(803) 737-6210 phone

Contact for annual statement information:
Timothy W. Campbell
(803) 737-6221 phone

Please note: Before data are requested from any source, it is advisable to telephone the source to confirm that the data sought are available in the time period desired. In addition, the cost and exact procedure for obtaining data are most easily explained in a telephone conversation.

South Dakota

The Department of Health conducts an annual hospital survey, from which discharge data and some financial data can be obtained. In addition to acute care facilities, the state collects data from psychiatric, rehabilitation, and children's facilities, as well as the Indian Health Service. Data are available on paper only, and the charge varies according to the data requested.

Requests for data should be directed to:

Barb Miller, Policy Analyst
South Dakota Department of Health
Center for Health Policy and Statistics
445 East Capitol Avenue
Pierre, SD 57501
(605) 773-3361 phone
(605) 773-5683 fax

Medicare cost reports can be requested from:

Blue Cross of Western Iowa and South Dakota
636 Grand Avenue, Station 28
Des Moines, IA 50309-2565
(515) 245-7538 phone
(515) 245-3965 fax

The state's hospital association can be contacted at:

South Dakota Hospital Association
3708 Brooks Place, Suite 1
Sioux Falls, SD 57106
(605) 361-2281 phone
(605) 361-5175 fax

Data contact person:

Garry Parry
(605) 361-5175 fax

Data are available on paper.

The state's insurance commissioner can be contacted at:

State Insurance Commissioner
Darla L. Lyon
Division of Insurance
Department of Commerce and Regulation
State of South Dakota
500 East Capitol Avenue
Pierre, SD 57501-5070
(605) 773-3563 phone
(605) 773-5369 fax

Contact for health insurance information:
Sherry Deaver
(605) 773-3563 phone

Contact for annual statement information:
Rose Marrington
(605) 773-3563 phone

Please note: Before data are requested from any source, it is advisable to telephone the source to confirm that the data sought are available in the time period desired. In addition, the cost and exact procedure for obtaining data are most easily explained in a telephone conversation.

Tennessee

Data are sorted by ICD-9 code and are available on magnetic tape. The charge varies according to the data requested. The Tennessee Department of Health also collects data on ambulatory surgery centers, home health agencies, and nursing homes.

Requests for data should be directed to:

Deborah Pauli
Tennessee Department of Health
Tennessee Tower, 8th Floor
312 8th Avenue North
Nashville, TN 37247-0340
(615) 532-7877 phone
(615) 532-7904 fax

Medicare cost reports can be requested from:

Blue Cross and Blue Shield of Tennessee
Provider Reimbursement Department
801 Pine Street
Chattanooga, TN 37402
(615) 755-5906 phone
(615) 752-7711 fax

The state's hospital association can be contacted at:

Tennessee Hospital Association
500 Interstate Boulevard, South
Nashville, TN 37210
(615) 256-8240 phone
(615) 242-4803 fax

The state's insurance commissioner can be contacted at:

State Insurance Commissioner
Allan S. Curtis
Department of Commerce and Insurance
State of Tennessee
Volunteer Plaza—500 James Robertson Parkway
Nashville, TN 37243-0565
(615) 741-2241 phone
(615) 741-4000 fax

Contact for health insurance information:
Howard Magill
(615) 741-2825 phone

Contact for annual statement information:
Don Spann
(615) 741-2637 phone

Please note: Before data are requested from any source, it is advisable to telephone the source to confirm that the data sought are available in the time period desired. In addition, the cost and exact procedure for obtaining data are most easily explained in a telephone conversation.

Texas

Hospital data are collected through the Cooperative TDH/AHA/THA Annual Survey of Texas Hospitals. Other data are obtained from various programs in the Texas Department of Health. Most data are available on paper; some data are available on diskette. Call for the price of standard reports and user-defined searches.

Requests for data should be directed to:

Dwayne Collins
Texas Department of Health
Bureau of State Health Data and Policy Analysis
1100 West 49th Street
Austin, TX 78756
(512) 458-7261 phone
(512) 458-7344 fax

Medicare cost reports can be requested from:

Blue Cross and Blue Shield of Texas, Inc.
901 South Central Expressway
Richardson, TX 75080
(214) 669-3900 phone
(214) 669-6060 fax

The state's hospital association can be contacted at:

Texas Hospital Association
6225 U.S. Highway 290 East
P.O. Box 15587
Austin, TX 78761-5587
(512) 465-1000 phone
(512) 465-1090 fax

The state's insurance commissioner can be contacted at:

State Insurance Commissioner
J. Robert Hunter
Texas Department of Insurance
P.O. Box 149104
Austin, TX 78714-9104
(512) 463-6169 phone
(512) 475-2005 fax

Contact for health insurance information:
Ladell Kielman
(512) 322-3409 phone

Contact for annual statement information:
Annual Statement Room
(512) 322-5002 phone

Please note: Before data are requested from any source, it is advisable to telephone the source to confirm that the data sought are available in the time period desired. In addition, the cost and exact procedure for obtaining data are most easily explained in a telephone conversation.

Utah

Call for specific reports available, data formats, and prices.
Requests for data should be directed to:

Denise Love
Office of Health Data Analysis
Utah Department of Health
288 North 1460 West
Salt Lake City, UT 84116
(801) 538-6689 phone
(801) 538-7053 fax

Medicare cost reports can be requested from:

Blue Cross and Blue Shield of Utah
Department #29
2455 Parley's Way
P.O. Box 30270
Salt Lake City, UT 84130
(801) 481-6198 phone
(801) 481-6994 fax

The state's hospital association can be contacted at:

Utah Association of Healthcare Providers
127 South 500 East, Suite 625
Salt Lake City, UT 84102
(801) 364-1515 phone
(801) 532-4806 fax

The state's insurance commissioner can be contacted at:

State Insurance Commissioner
Robert E. Wilcox
Department of Insurance
State of Utah
State Office Building, Room 3110
Salt Lake City, UT 84114-1201
(801) 538-3800 phone
(801) 538-3829 fax

Contact for health insurance information:
DeLone Cates
(801) 538-3861 phone

Contact for annual statement information:
Rene Kidd
(801) 538-3813 phone

Please note: Before data are requested from any source, it is advisable to telephone the source to confirm that the data sought are available in the time period desired. In addition, the cost and exact procedure for obtaining data are most easily explained in a telephone conversation.

Vermont

Facility utilization data are provided from the Division of Public Health Analysis and Policy by DRG or ICD-9 code. Data are available on magnetic tape or diskette in either standard format or user-defined searches. Contact the Division for prices.

Requests for data should be directed to:

John Gauthier
Research and Statistics Analyst
Department of Health
Division of Public Health Analysis and Policy
108 Cherry Street
P.O. Box 70
Burlington, VT 05402
(802) 863-7300 phone
(802) 863-7425 fax

Requests for financial data should be directed to:

Michael Davis, Executive Director
Vermont Hospital Data Council
Health Care Authority
89 Main Street, Drawer 20
Montpelier, VT 05620-3601
(802) 828-2900 phone
(802) 828-2949 fax

Medicare cost reports can be requested from:

New Hampshire–Vermont Health Service
3000 Goffs Falls Road
Manchester, NH 03111-0001
(603) 695-7000 phone
(603) 695-7095 fax

The state's hospital association can be contacted at:

Vermont Hospital Association
148 Main Street
Montpelier, VT 05602
(802) 223-3461 phone
(802) 223-0364 fax

The state's insurance commissioner can be contacted at:

State Insurance Commissioner
Elizabeth R. Costle
Division of Insurance
Department of Banking, Insurance, and Securities
89 Main Street, Drawer 20
Montpelier, VT 05620-3101
(802) 828-3301 phone
(802) 828-3306 fax

Contact for health insurance information:
Lyle Moulton
(802) 828-3301 phone

Contact for annual statement information:
Mitch Fried
(802) 828-4850 phone

Please note: Before data are requested from any source, it is advisable to telephone the source to confirm that the data sought are available in the time period desired. In addition, the cost and exact procedure for obtaining data are most easily explained in a telephone conversation.

Virginia

Inpatient data are available by ICD-9 code on paper, magnetic tape, and diskette. The charge varies according to the data requested.

Requests for state-level data should be directed to:

Michael Lundberg
Virginia Health Information
The Plantation House
1108 East Main Street, Suite 1201
Richmond, VA 23219
(804) 643-5573 phone
(804) 643-5375 fax

Ann McGee
Virginia Health Services Cost Review Council
805 East Broad Street, 6th Floor
Richmond, VA 23219
(804) 786-6371 phone
(804) 371-0284 fax

Other requests for data should be directed to:

Calvin Reynolds, Statistical Analyst
Virginia State Department of Health
P.O. Box 1000
Richmond, VA 23208-1000
(804) 786-3698 phone
(804) 371-4800 fax

Medicare cost reports can be requested from:

Provider Audit and Reimbursement
Trigon Blue Cross Blue Shield
2015 Staples Mill Road
Mail Drop 43D-Dox 27401
Richmond, VA 23279
(804) 354 2260 phone
(804) 354-2232 fax
or
Department of Medical Assistance Service
600 East Broad Street, Suite 1300
Richmond, VA 23219
(804) 786-7933 phone
(804) 225-4512 fax

The state's hospital association can be contacted at:

Virginia Hospital Association
P.O. Box 31394
Richmond, VA 23294
(804) 747-8600 phone
(804) 965-0475 fax

Data contact person:

David L. Moore
Director of Data Services
Virginia Hospital Association
P.O. Box 31394
Richmond, VA 23237

Data are not made available to the general public.

The state's insurance commissioner can be contacted at:

State Insurance Commissioner
Steven T. Foster
State Corporation Commission/Bureau of Insurance
Commonwealth of Virginia
P.O. Box 1157
Richmond, VA 23209
(804) 371-9694 phone
(804) 371-9873 fax

Contact for health insurance information:
Gerald A. Milsky
(804) 371-9074 phone

Contact for annual statement information:
Edward J. Buyalos, Jr.
(804) 371-9637 phone

Please note: Before data are requested from any source, it is advisable to telephone the source to confirm that the data sought are available in the time period desired. In addition, the cost and exact procedure for obtaining data are most easily explained in a telephone conversation.

Washington

Data are available either by DRG or ICD-9 codes on paper, magnetic tape, or diskette. The charge varies according to the data requested.

Washington participates in an Agency for Health Care Policy and Research project called the Healthcare Cost and Utilization Project (HCUP-3). HCUP-3 has created the State Inpatient Database, which provides comparable inpatient data for 12 states: Arizona, California, Colorado, Florida, Illinois, Iowa, Massachusetts, New Jersey, New York, Pennsylvania, Washington, and Wisconsin. Each state has established policies and procedures for gaining access to state data. Requests related to the Washington HCUP-3 State Inpatient Database should be directed to:

Hank Brown
Washington State Department of Health
Office of Hospital and Patient Data Systems
1102 SE Quince Street
P.O. Box 47811
Olympia, WA 98504-7811
(360) 705-6007 phone
(360) 705-6020 fax

If information is needed regarding the HCUP-3 project in general, please contact the Agency for Health Care Policy and Research, Division of Provider Studies, Center for Intramural Research, (301) 594-1410 (phone), (301) 594-2314 (fax), hcupSID@cghsir.ahcpr.gov (via Internet).

Requests for state-level data should be directed to:

Vicki Hohner
Washington State Department of Health
P.O. Box 47811
Olympia, WA 98504-7811
(360) 705-6027 phone
(360) 705-6020 fax
vkh0303@hub.doh.wa.gov via Internet

Other requests for data should be directed to:

Larry Hettick, Financial Analysis Supervisor
Health Information Division
Office of Hospital and Patient Data Systems
1102 SE Quince Street
P.O. Box 47811
Olympia, WA 98504-7811
(360) 705-6014 phone
(360) 705-6020 fax

Requests for additional DRG information should be directed to:

Diana M.Johnson
CHARS Manager
Washington State Department of Health
Office of Hospital and Patient Data Systems
1102 SE Quince Street
P.O. Box 47811
Olympia, WA 98504-7811
(360) 705-6011 phone
(360) 705-6020 fax

Medicare cost reports can be requested from:

Epidemiology and Health Statistics
Office of Hospital and Patient Data Systems
P.O. Box 47811
Olympia, WA 98504-7811
(360) 705-6014 phone
(360) 705-6020 fax

The state's hospital association can be contacted at:

Washington State Hospital Association
300 Elliott Avenue West, Suite 300
Seattle, WA 98119-4118
(206) 281-7211 phone
(206) 283-6122 fax

The state's insurance commissioner can be contacted at:

State Insurance Commissioner
Deborah Senn
Office of Insurance Commissioner
State of Washington
P.O. Box 40255
Olympia, WA 98504-0255
(360) 753-7300 phone
(360) 586-3535 fax

Contact for health insurance information:
Janis LaFlash
(360) 753-4214 phone

Contact for annual statement information:
John Woodall
(360) 753-7303 phone

Please note: Before data are requested from any source, it is advisable to telephone
the source to confirm that the data sought are available in the time period desired.
In addition, the cost and exact procedure for obtaining data are most easily
explained in a telephone conversation.

West Virginia

Data are collated by DRG and are available on paper, magnetic tape, and diskette. The charge varies according to the data requested and the format. The Health Care Cost Review Authority also collects utilization and financial data on ambulatory surgical centers and skilled nursing facilities.

Requests for data should be directed to:

Ray Shingler
West Virginia Health Care Cost Review Authority
100 Dee Drive, Suite 201
Charleston, WV 25311-1692
(304) 558-7000 phone
(304) 558-7001 fax

Medicare cost reports can be requested from:

Mountain State Blue Cross and Blue Shield
700 Market Street
Parkersburg, WV 26102
(304) 424-7700 phone
(304) 424-7730 fax

The state's hospital association can be contacted at:

West Virginia Hospital Association
600 D Street, Second Level
South Charleston, WV 25303
(304) 744-9842 phone
(304) 744-9889 fax

The state's insurance commissioner can be contacted at:

State Insurance Commissioner
Hanley C. Clark
Department of Insurance
State of West Virginia
2019 Washington Street East
P.O. Box 50540
Charleston, WV 25305-0504
(304) 558-3354 phone
(304) 558-1610 fax

Contact for health insurance information:
Jerry W. Gladwell
(304) 558-2094 phone

Contact for annual statement information:
John M. Collins
(304) 558-2100 phone

Please note: Before data are requested from any source, it is advisable to telephone the source to confirm that the data sought are available in the time period desired. In addition, the cost and exact procedure for obtaining data are most easily explained in a telephone conversation.

Wisconsin

The Office of Health Care Information collects ongoing data from the facilities on a quarterly basis. A number of collated data reports are available on paper. A product guide is available that describes the data collected, standard reports done, and formats. New data sets become available to the public approximately four months after the end of each calendar quarter. Records of individual inpatient discharges, hospital-based outpatient surgeries, or surgeries performed at freestanding ambulatory surgery centers can be supplied on computer media in a number of different formats including magnetic tape in ASCII or EBCDIC formats, or on diskette in ASCII format. Data are available either in standard report formats or tailored to the user's specifications. The charge varies according to the data requested. Contact the office for specific prices.

Requests for data should be directed to:

Trudy A. Karlson, Director
State of Wisconsin
Office of the Commissioner of Insurance
Office of Health Care Information
121 East Wilson, Box 7984
Madison, WI 53707-7984
(608) 266-7568 phone
(608) 264-9881 fax

Wisconsin participates in an Agency for Health Care Policy and Research project called the Healthcare Cost and Utilization Project (HCUP-3). HCUP-3 has created the State Inpatient Database, which provides comparable inpatient data for 12 states: Arizona, California, Colorado, Florida, Illinois, Iowa, Massachusetts, New Jersey, New York, Pennsylvania, Washington, and Wisconsin. Each state has established policies and procedures for gaining access to state data. Requests related to the Wisconsin HCUP-3 State Inpatient Database should be directed to:

Judith Nugent
State of Wisconsin
Office of the Commissioner of Insurance
Office of Health Care Information
121 East Wilson, Box 7984
Madison, WI 53707-7984
(608) 266-2863 phone
(608) 264-9881 fax

If information is needed regarding the HCUP-3 project in general, please contact the Agency for Health Care Policy and Research, Division of Provider Studies, Center for Intramural Research, (301) 594-1410 (phone), (301) 594-2314 (fax), hcupSID@cghsir.ahcpr.gov (via Internet).

Medicare cost reports can be requested from:

Blue Cross and Blue Shield United of Wisconsin
P.O. Box 2025
Milwaukee, WI 53201
(414) 224-6100 phone
(414) 226-5040 fax

The state's hospital association can be contacted at:

Wisconsin Hospital Association
5721 Odana Road
Madison, WI 53719-1289
(608) 274-1820 phone
(608) 274-8554 fax

The state's insurance commissioner can be contacted at:

State Insurance Commissioner
Josephine W. Musser
Office of the Commissioner of Insurance
State of Wisconsin
P.O. Box 7873
Madison, WI 53707-7873
(608) 266-3585 phone
(608) 266-9935 fax

Contact for health insurance information:
Complaint and Central Services Section
(608) 266-0103 phone

Contact for annual statement information:
Yvonne Sherry
(608) 266-0091 phone

Please note: Before data are requested from any source, it is advisable to telephone the source to confirm that the data sought are available in the time period desired. In addition, the cost and exact procedure for obtaining data are most easily explained in a telephone conversation.

Wyoming

All hospital data are collected and analyzed by the Wyoming Hospital Association. Both the Wyoming Department of Health and the Wyoming Hospital Association state that data are released to Wyoming hospitals only.

Requests for data should be directed to:

Donna Andersen, Administrative Assistant
Wyoming Hospital Association
P.O. Box 5539
Cheyenne, WY 82003
(307) 632-9344 phone
(307) 632-9347 fax

Medicare cost reports can be requested from:

Blue Cross and Blue Shield of Wyoming
4000 House Avenue
P.O. Box 2266
Cheyenne, WY 82001
(307) 634-1393 phone
(307) 778-8582 fax

The state's hospital association can be contacted at:

Donna Andersen, Administrative Assistant
Wyoming Hospital Association
P.O. Box 5539
Cheyenne, WY 82003
(307) 632-9344 phone
(307) 632-9347 fax

The state's insurance commissioner can be contacted at:

State Insurance Commissioner
John P. McBride
Department of Insurance
State of Wyoming
Herscher Building
122 West 25th Street, 3rd East
Cheyenne, WY 82002-0440
(307) 777-7401 phone
(307) 777-5895 fax

Contact for health insurance information:
Mark Pring
(307) 777-6888 phone

Contact for annual statement information:
Audrey Hayes
(307) 777-7318 phone

Please note: Before data are requested from any source, it is advisable to telephone the source to confirm that the data sought are available in the time period desired. In addition, the cost and exact procedure for obtaining data are most easily explained in a telephone conversation.

Appendix E

Electronic Access to Data

Paper is by far the most common format for health care data transmission today. However, given the long lead time for producing publications, the time consumed by transporting paper data from point A to point B, and the necessity of sifting through endless pages to extract a few pertinent facts, electronic data are becoming more and more attractive. The rapidly changing nature of the health care field makes quick dissemination and uptake of relevant data a necessity.

Fortunately, the fastest-growing source of health care data today is as close as your personal computer and modem. Data on every facet of health care from AIDS to X rays can be found with the right combination of keystrokes. Data formats range from the familiar magnetic tapes and diskettes to CD-ROMs and the challenging world of the Internet, with its bewildering array of Webs, WAISs, Gophers, and MOSAICs.

A word of caution is in order, however. It is easier to become inundated with electronic information than it is to become buried in paper. A hard disk will contain much more information than even a large desk stacked deep with journals and reports. Be as selective in your dealings with electronic information as you would in subscribing to paper journals.

Forms of Electronic Data and Hardware Requirements

The following list of resources touches on all the forms of electronic data: "off-line" media such as magnetic tapes, diskettes, and CD-ROMs, and "on-line" data such as databases, bulletin boards, catalogues, user groups, list servers, and electronic publications. Paper references that can help direct readers to electronic data are also provided. As a rule, data available on diskette are targeted to a particular use; for example, state inpatient hospital utilization statistics. *Databases* are large collections of data that are related in some coherent manner, for example, CANCERLIT contains references to publications all dealing with some aspect of cancer. *Bulletin boards* are just that, electronic listings of data available or pointers to discussion groups. Health care bulletin boards are usually focused on one aspect of health care, such as AIDS or health care management. *Catalogues* are the electronic equivalent of library card catalogues. They usually list the publications available from some institution or agency and provide the same information one would expect to find on a card in a card catalogue. Some catalogues (for example, MEDLINE) allow people to order the publications they are interested in. *User groups* are the electronic equivalent of roundtable discussions, in which members may pose questions and receive answers, usually to some health care–focused questions. *List servers* (for example, NITS FAX Direct) can be thought of as a type of clipping service in which people may indicate their interest in receiving information on specific topics.

With the exception of the magnetic tape, the hardware required to access these resources is commonly found in offices: either a 386 (or preferably a 486) IBM-compatible PC with a CD-ROM drive, 4 (or more) megabytes of memory, a hard drive, and a modem capable of transmitting at 2400 baud (at a minimum). A Macintosh computer and modem with the same capability will also work. Either computer will need some type of communications software that allows the computer to "look like" a dumb terminal.

Internet Access and Resources

Although some of the agencies listed in this appendix have access numbers for dialing in directly, the easiest way to access the greatest range of resources is to use the Internet. Although the Internet has been primarily used as a research and academic tool, it is becoming the "information superhighway" for those in the health care field. In the past, access to the Internet has been limited to individuals who hold positions in government or to those associated with an institution of higher learning, but it is now possible to access the full range of Internet services through commercial services.

Several of the larger commercially available communications networks such as CompuServe, Prodigy, and America Online allow access to the electronic mail portion of the Internet. This enables users to send and receive messages from anyone who has an Internet address anywhere in the world, all for whatever the commercial service charges (appreciably less than long-distance telephone charges). The full range of Internet services (that is, accessing remote databases and catalogues and copying and receiving files) is only available (at the time of this writing) through Delphi, a commercial service. After signing up with the service, you select a "user ID" that becomes your "name" on the Internet. After that, where you go and what you find out is limited only by your persistence.

There are, unfortunately, no Yellow Pages to the Internet that list all possible user IDs or services and data that one could access. Indeed, one of the most useful and yet frustrating aspects of the Internet is that the same resource is available via a number of different pathways, some of which even are free. Navigating to an Internet resource has been likened to finding a particular house in a city. There are multiple streets one could take to reach that destination, but some routes have advantages over others. Although there is no single comprehensive guide that lists all the navigating commands and where to use them, a multitude of commercially available publications do address certain aspects of navigating the Internet. One useful guide for beginners is *The Internet Companion* (Reading, MA: Addison-Wesley, 1993) by T. LaQuey.

An "Internet Health Science Resource List" is maintained by Lee Hancock, an educational technologist at the University of Kansas Medical Center. This list contains more than 200 printed pages of references to bulletin boards, databases, user discussion groups, and health sciences "Gophers" (software designed to organize access to data on the Internet). To obtain an electronic copy of the list, send $20.00 and a formatted diskette to Lee Hancock, 3580 Rainbow Boulevard #826, Kansas City, KS 66103.

Electronic Resources

The following list is a sample of some of the electronic resources available. Addresses and telephone or fax numbers not listed here can be found in the section entitled "Information for Ordering Studies and Reports" at the end of appendix F. The last entry listed before the order or publication number is the source.

Bulletin Boards

CancerNet: This service lets the user request information from the National Cancer Institute. Information includes the fact sheets on various cancers and citations and abstracts from the CANCERLIT database. For access, e-mail to cancernet@icicb.nci.nih.gov.

Federal Bulletin Board: Self-service access to government information in electronic formats. Accessible via modem by dialing (202) 512-1387 (modem settings 8N1, full duplex) or telnet to Federal.bbs.gop.gov 3001 on the

Internet. Phone (202) 512-1530 for rates and further information, or (202) 512-1262 to fax information.

NAPHS Online (National Association of Psychiatric Health Systems): An electronic communications system for NAPHS members providing computer access to a full range of mental health information, including legislative and regulatory information, a mental health library, and a "members only" bulletin board. The fee is $265.00 per year. Call (202) 393-6700 for details.

CD-ROMs

HCFA's Laws and Regulations Manual CD-ROM: 1994; $274.00. List ID HCLRM, Government Printing Office.

Databases

AHA Annual Survey of Hospitals Data Base: 1993; American Hospital Association, catalog no. C-083394 tape (EBCDIC), catalog no. C-083494 (ASCII), catalog no. C-083594 3-1/2-inch diskette. Call for prices.

CINAHL: A nursing, allied health, and health education database available from SilverPlatter Information, Inc., (800) 343-0064.

FEDRIP (Federal Research in Progress) Database: Offered through NTIS, this database provides information about federal health care research currently in progress, allowing access to information before technical reports or journal literature becomes available. Call (703) 487-4650 and request PR-847/CAU for a free search guide. The database may be searched through Dialog, (800) 334-2564, Knowledge Express, (215) 293-9712, and NERAC Inc., (203) 872-7000.

FedWorld: A database of government databases. An electronic access point to locate, order, and acquire U.S. and foreign government information. Connect directly via modem at (703) 321-8020. Set your modem for Parity = NONE, Data Bits = 8, Stop Bits = 1 (N-8-1) with a terminal emulation of either ANSI or VT-100. FedWorld accommodates speeds up to 9600 baud. To connect to FedWorld via Internet, telnet to: fedworld.gov.

HealthPLAN-CD: A database produced by the National Library of Medicine and the American Hospital Association that addresses issues such as insurance and regulation of medical facilities, available from SilverPlatter Information, Inc., (800) 343-0064.

MEDLARS: The National Library of Medicine group of databases. For on-line access information, e-mail to Management Section: mms@nlm.nih.gov.

MEDLARS databases include:

AIDSLINE: A comprehensive source for clinical and research aspects of AIDS, epidemiology, and health policy issues. Contains information from journal articles, meeting papers, symposia, dissertations, books, government reports, and audiovisuals from 1980 to the present.

BIOETHICSLINE: The database contains information specific to ethical issues in medicine. Information is drawn from numerous sources that include journals, court decisions, and legal materials. Information covers data from 1973 to the present.

HST (Health Services/Technology Assessment Research): An on-line database that provides access to published literature of health services research. Health services research (HSR) is the study of the scientific basis and management of health services and their effect on access, quality, and cost of health care. HST is available on the NLM computer system 24 hours a day and may be searched using GRATEFUL MED. For information on accessing or obtaining NLM user code, contact:
MEDLARS Management Section
National Library of Medicine
8600 Rockville Pike
Bethesda, MD 20894
(800) 638-8480 phone
mms@nlm.nih.gov via Internet

MEDLINE: Contains abstracts to articles from 3,500 journal titles with data as far back as 1982. For access information, e-mail to ref@nlm.nih.gov.

A software package called GRATEFUL MED is available for $30.00 and provides a menu-driven aid for searching many of the NLM databases. In addition, an enhancement called LOANSOME DOC allows the user to order copies of articles of interest from participating medical libraries. For information about both programs, e-mail to: gmhelp@medserv.nlm.nih.gov.

NTIS (National Technical Information Service) Bibliographic Database: Summaries of information from 1964 to the present. Information is available as reports, videos, software, and data files. On-line access to the database is provided by BRS; CISTI; DIALOG DATA-STAR; DIALOG Information Services; European Space Agency/Research Institute (in Italy);

NERAC, Inc.; ORBIT/QUESTEL, Inc.; and STN International. (See the end of appendix F for addresses and telephone and fax numbers.) Intensive users of the database may wish to purchase a copy of the database on CD-ROM.

NTIS Database on CD-ROM: DIALOG Information Services offers records from 1980 to the present. SilverPlatter Information, Inc., offers it from 1983 to the present. Both services update the CD-ROM quarterly.

NTIS FAX Direct: NTIS distributes directly to your fax machine free subject-specific lists of the scientific, technical, and business titles requested most often by NTIS customers. Call (703) 487-4099 from any Touch-Tone® phone to be connected to the computer. Press "1" to get the latest master list of subject-specific lists: *Guide to NTIS Most Frequently Requested Titles.* After you have the list, enter the identifying code numbers by phone to request individual lists.

NTIS Training: NTIS offers on-line and CD-ROM training. For information, call the NTIS Online Training Coordinator at (703) 487-4078.

Diskettes

Health, United States, 1992: Set of ten 3-1/2-inch PC diskettes, U.S. government statistical review, 1993, $37.00; Government Printing Office, stock no. 017-022-01250-2.

Hospital Data by Geographic Area for Aged Medicare Beneficiaries: Selected Diagnostic Groups, 1986 (Procedures V01 Segments 1–4): Diskette, $250.00; National Technical Information Service, order no. PB91-507384CBA (HCFA).

Hospital Data by Geographic Area for Aged Medicare Beneficiaries: Selected Procedures, 1986 (Procedures V02 Segments 1–3): Diskette, $195.00; National Technical Information Service, order no. PB91-507392CBA (HCFA).

Measuring Prices of Medicare Physician Services: 1985–1988: Diskette, $90.00; National Technical Information Service, order no. PB92-504299CBA (HCFA).

Physician's Practice Cost & Income Survey (PPCIS) Data Base System, 1983–1985: Diskette, $195.00; National Technical Information Service, order no. PB89-106975CBA (HCFA).

Rehospitalization by Geographic Area for Aged Medicare Beneficiaries: Selected Procedures, 1986–1987, Volume 3 Table Data: Diskette, $90.00; National Technical Information Service, order no. PB91-507418CBA (HCFA).

Magnetic Tape

Income and Assets Supplement to the Medicare Current Beneficiary 1991 Round 1 Public Use Release: Magnetic tape, $240.00; National Technical Information Service, order no. PB93-505451CBA (HCFA).

Medicare Current Beneficiary Survey 191 Round 1 Public Use Release: Magnetic tape, $480.00; National Technical Information Service, order no. PB93-500262CBA (HCFA).

Medicare Current Beneficiary Survey 1992 Access to Care: Magnetic tape, $480.00; National Technical Information Service, order no. PB94-500022CBA (HCFA).

Physician's Practice Cost and Income Survey, 1988: Magnetic tape, $240.00; National Technical Information Service, order no. PB92-504224CBA (HCFA).

On-Line Journals

FaxAlert: Automatic notification of activity of interest to subscriber to US HealthLink, $10.00 per month; Medical Software Products, order no. 245-03.

US HealthLink-On-Line Medical Information Network: I.E.I. Network, Inc., $35.00 per month; Medical Software Products, order no. 245-01.

Software

Automated AMH (Accreditation Manual for Hospitals): 1994, $495.00; JCAHO, order code EMH-94 S.

CDC WONDER: A DOS-based product that creates a link between the Centers for Disease Control and the user. Access is currently only by modem and not directly via the Internet. For information about registration, contact:
Dan Rosen
Public Health Information Systems Branch
Centers for Disease Control and Prevention
4770 Buford Highway
MS F-51
Atlanta, GA 30341-3724
(404) 488-7521 phone
(404) 488-7593 fax
dhr0@opsirm8.em.cdc.gov

Medical Software Reviews: Healthcare Computing Publications, $75.00 per year; Medical Software Products, order no. 205-01.

Score 100: A Tool for Predicting Survey Outcomes: 1993, $1,495.00; JCAHO, order code SC94H.

User Groups

HEALTHMGMT: A discussion group for those in health care management and health service organizations. The electronic discussion list is for the Health Administration Division of the Academy of Management. For access, e-mail to chimera.sph.umn.edu.

Paper References

Clinical Data Management: $189.00 per year; Aspen Publishers.

Data Collection Organization Effects in the National Medical Expenditure Survey: 1990; National Center for Health Statistics, order no. OM 91-0503.

Data Files from the 1987 National Medical Expenditure Survey. Information of Public Use Tapes and Other NMES-2 Data Available to the Public: 1993; Agency for Health Care Policy and Research, order no. 94-0011.

Health Maintenance Organizations—Information Systems: 1993, $15.00; MGMA, order no. 3477.

Appendix F

Selected Studies and Reports

This appendix lists studies and reports that would typically be of interest to hospital planning and marketing personnel. The last entry for a particular report (before the order or publication number) is the source of the report. To find the address and telephone number for a source of a publication, see the final section of this appendix, Information for Ordering Studies and Reports. This section also provides expansions for the abbreviations of company names used in this appendix. The main categories of studies and reports listed in this appendix are as follows:

- Cost of Health Care
- Directories and Basic Reference Books
- Effectiveness and Efficiency of Procedures and Technology
- Health Care Utilization
- Health Insurance
- Hospital Management: General Management Information
- Hospital Management: Specific Hospital Service Lines
- Managed Care
- Physician Supply
- Statistical Data and Surveys (Compilations)

Cost of Health Care

Administrative Costs and the Debate About U.S. Health System Reform: A Review of the Literature, 1994, $15.00; AMA.

Annual Expenses and Sources of Payment for Health Care Services, 1992; Agency for Health Care Planning and Research, order no. 93-0007.

Are Fee-for-Service Costs Increasing Faster Than HMO Costs?, 1985, $4.00; RAND Corporation, order no. N-2364-HHS.

The Concentration of Health Expenditures: An Update, 1992; Agency for Health Care Policy and Research, order no. 93-0031.

Costs of AIDS and Other HIV Infections: Review of the Estimates, 1987; Office of Technology Assessment Health Program.

Cost Survey: 1993 Report Based on 1992 Data, 1993, $200.00; MGMA, order no. 3334.

Cost Survey: 1994 Report Based on 1993 Data, 1994, $210.00; MGMA, order no. 4042.

The Demand for Prescription Drugs as a Function of Cost-Sharing, 1985, $4.00; RAND Corporation, order no. N-2278-HHS.

Determinants of Hospital Costs: Outputs, Inputs, and Regulation in the 1980's, 1991, $16.50; The Urban Institute, ISBN no. 0-87766-552-4.

The Effects of Cost Sharing and Physician Specialty on the Costs of Office-Based Medical Care, 1988, $10.00; RAND Corporation, order no. P-7547-RGS.

The Effect of Cost Sharing on the Use of Antibiotics in Ambulatory Care: Results from a Population-Based Randomized Controlled Trial, 1987, $4.00; RAND Corporation, order no. N-2712-HHS/RC.

The Effects of Hospital Competition and the Medicare PPS Program on Hospital Cost Behavior in California, 1988, $4.00; RAND Corporation, order no. N-3049-HHS/PMT.

Factors Contributing to the Health Care Cost Problem, 1994, $15.00; AMA.

Fee-for-Service Health Care Expenditures: Evidence of Selection Effects among Subscribers Who Choose HMOs, 1986, $7.50; RAND Corporation, order no. R-3341-HHS.

An Inconsistent Picture: A Compilation of Analyses of Economic Impacts of Competing Approaches to Health Care Reform by Experts and Stakeholders, 1993, $8.00; Government Printing Office, stock no. 052-003-01327-4.

Informing Consumers about Health Care Costs: A Review and Research Agenda, 1985, $7.50; RAND Corporation, order no. R-3262-HCFA.

Medicaid: Changes in Drug Prices Paid by HMO's and Hospitals Since Enactment of Rebate Provisions, 1993; General Accounting Office (HRD-93-43).

Spotlight on Health Cost Management, 1993, $10.00; National Association of Manufacturers.

Use and Cost of Health Services: Effect of Health Insurance and Other Factors, 1993; Agency for Health Care Planning and Research, order no. 93-0121.

Directories and Basic Reference Books

General References

AHA Guide to the Health Care Field, 1994, $195.00; AHA, catalog no. C-010094.

The Directory of U.S. Hospitals, 1994, $219.00 (paper), $899.00 (diskette); Health Care Investment Analysts.

Health Reports (1990–92), 1992; General Accounting Office (HRD-93-38).

Health Reports (1988–92), 1992; General Accounting Office (HRD-93-66).

Hospital Software Sourcebook, 1993, $125.00; Aspen Publishers.

1993 National Health Directory, 1993, $89.00; Aspen Publishers.

103rd Congress Directory, 1994, $7.00; National Association of Manufacturers.

The Prevention Index, 1993 Report on the Nation's Health, 1993; The Prevention Index.

Readiness for Reform—An Analysis of 16 U.S. Metropolitan Areas and Their Preparedness for Health Care Reform, 1994; Northwestern National Life Insurance Companies.

Statistical Abstract of the United States 1993, $29.00 (paper), $34.00 (hardcover); National Technical Information Service, order no. PB92-169069/CAU or PB92-169051/CAU.

Health Insurance and Managed Care

Note: For further information on this topic, see the main headings for Health Insurance and Managed Care, as well as the subheading under Statistical Data and Surveys (Compilations).

The Guide to the Managed Care Industry, 1994, $199.00 (paper), $899.00 (diskette); Health Care Investment Analysts.

Health Maintenance Organizations, 1994, $425.00; SMG Marketing Group.

Insurance Department Directory, 1994, $25.00; National Association of Insurance Commissioners.

The Managed Care Assembly (MCA) Directory: 1993 Report Based on 1992 Data, 1993, $73.00; MGMA, order no. 4049.

National HMO Directory, HMO Industry Report, Regional HMO Market Analysis, 1994, $315.00; InterStudy Publications.

NWNL 1994 State Health Rankings, 1994; Northwestern National Life Insurance Companies.

Preferred Provider Organizations, 1994, $425.00; SMG Marketing Group.

Specific Disciplines

Ambulatory (Urgent) Care Centers, 1994, $425.00; SMG Marketing Group.

The Directory of Nursing Homes, 1994, $249.00 (paper), call for electronic media price; Health Care Investment Analysts.

The Directory of Retirement Facilities, 1994, $249.00 (paper), call for electronic media price; Health Care Investment Analysts.

The Guide to the Nursing Home Industry, 1994, $249.00 (paper), $599.00 (diskette); Health Care Investment Analysts.

Medical Group Practices: 5+ Physicians, 1994, $425.00; SMG Marketing Group.

The Directory of Medical Rehabilitation Programs, 1994, $195.00 (paper), $699.00 (tape or diskette); Health Care Investment Analysts.

NAPHS Guide to Mental Health and Substance Abuse Resources, 1994, $15.00; National Association of Psychiatric Health Systems, item no. GMH.

NAPHS Membership Roster (National Association of Psychiatric Health Systems), 1994, $15.00; National Association of Psychiatric Health Systems, item no. ROS.

Outpatient Surgery Centers, 1994, $425.00; SMG Marketing Group.

Utilization Management Coordinator's Roster, 1994, $10.00; National Association of Psychiatric Health Systems, item no. UMR.

Effectiveness and Efficiency of Procedures and Technology

Analysis of Medically Unnecessary Inpatient Services, 1994; Milliman & Robertson.

Cost and Effectiveness of Cervical Cancer Screening, 1990; National Technical Information Service, order no. PB90-166018.

Cost and Effectiveness of Cholesterol Screening in the Elderly, 1989; National Technical Information Service, order no. PB89-224638.

Cost and Effectiveness of Colorectal Cancer Screening in the Elderly, 1990; National Technical Information Service, order no. PB90-166018.

Hip Fracture Outcomes in People Age 50 and Over: Mortality, Service Use, Expenditures, and Long-Term Functional Impairment, 1993; National Technical Information Service, order no. PB94-107653.

National Ambulatory Medical Care Survey: 1991 Summary, 1993; Advance Data Reports, PHS 93-1250, CDC.

Technology and Aging in America, Biological Applications Program (BA-264), 1985; National Technical Information Service, order no. PB86-116514.

Health Care Utilization

Health Care Utilization Analyses from the National Hospital Discharge Survey

Note: The National Hospital Discharge Survey is a continuous nationwide survey of inpatient utilization of acute care hospitals conducted by the National Center for Health Statistics. Survey data are abstracted from sampled medical records of inpatients discharged from a national sample of non–Federal short-stay hospitals. Although the survey is nationwide, it allows analysis at the census division level [regional levels as of 1988]. Beginning in 1979, ICD-9-CM was used to code diagnoses and procedures.

Detailed Diagnoses and Procedures, National Hospital Discharge Survey, 1991, 1992, $19.00; Government Printing Office, stock no. 017-022-01248-1, CDC.

Long-Stay Patients in Short-Stay Hospitals, 1993; Advance Data Report, PHS93-1250, CDC.

National Ambulatory Medical Care Survey: 1989 Summary, 1992, $10.00; Government Printing Office, stock no. 017-022-01155-7, CDC.

National Hospital Discharge Survey: Annual Summary, 1991, 1992, $6.00; Government Printing Office, stock no. 017-022-001219-7.

Specialty Utilization Data from the National Center for Health Statistics

Health Characteristics of Large Metropolitan Statistical Areas: United States, 1988–89, 1993, $6.50; Government Printing Office, stock no. 017-022-01221-9, CDC.

Health Conditions Among the Currently Employed: United States, 1988, 1993, $5.00; Government Printing Office, stock no. 017-022-01206-5, CDC.

Health, United States, 1993, 1993, $19.00; Government Printing Office, stock no. 017-022-01252-9, CDC.

National Health Expenditures, 1990, 1990; Office of National Health Statistics.

National Hospital Ambulatory Medical Care Survey: 1992 Outpatient Department Summary, 1994; PHS 94-1250, CDC.

Office Visits to General Surgeons 1989–90, National Ambulatory Medical Care Survey, 1993; Advance Data Report PHS 93-1250, CDC.

Projections of National Health Expenditures through the Year 2000, 1990; Office of National Health Statistics.

Utilization Reports and Statistical Summaries

Aggregated Claims Series: Vol. 1, Codebook for Fee-for-Service Annual Expenditures and Visit Counts, 1986, $7.50; RAND Corporation, order no. N-2360/1-HHS.

Aggregated Claims Series: Vol. 2, Codebooks for Fee-for-Service Visits— Outpatient, Inpatient, and Dental, 1986, $15.00; RAND Corporation, order no. N-2360/2.

Aggregated Claims Series: Vol. 3, Codebooks for Fee-for-Service Treatment Episodes and Annual Episode Counts, 1986, $10.00; RAND Corporation, order no. N-2360/3-HHS.

Aggregated Claims Series: Vol. 4, Codebooks for Health Maintenance Organization and Seattle Fee-for-Service Visits—Outpatient and Inpatient, 1986, $15.00; RAND Corporation, order no. N-2360/4-HHS.

Aggregated Claims Series: Vol. 5, Codebooks for Health Maintenance Organization and Seattle Fee-for-Service Annual Expenditures and Visit Counts, 1986, $10.00; RAND Corporation, order no. N-2360/5-HHS.

Choice under Uncertainty and the Demand for Health Insurance, 1986, $4.00; RAND Corporation, order no. N-2516-HHS.

Codebooks for Insurance Preference Files: Relation between Expense Limit and Premium, 1986, $7.50; RAND Corporation, order no. N-2508-HHS.

The 50 Most Frequent Diagnosis Related Groups (DRG's), Diagnoses, and Procedures: Statistics by Hospital Size and Location, 1990; Agency for Health Care Policy and Research, order no. PHS 90-3465.

Geographic Variations in Physician Service Utilization and Implications for Health Reform, 1993, $8.50; The Urban Institute, working paper no. 2352.

HCUP-2 Project Overview, 1988; Agency for Health Care Policy and Research, order no. PHS 88-3428.

HIE Reference Series: Vol. 3, User's Guide to HIE Data, 1987, $15.00; RAND Corporation, order no. N-2349/3-HHS.

The Impact of Cost Sharing on Emergency Department Use, 1985, $4.00; RAND Corporation, order no. N-2376-HHS.

1985 National Nursing Home Survey Utilization Data—Transactions 1988–89–90 Reports of Mortality, Morbidity and Other Experience, 1991, $50.00; Long-Term Care Experience Committee, Society of Actuaries.

Patterns of Hospital Utilization among Privately Insured Patients, 1980–1986, 1990; Agency for Health Care Policy and Research, order no. OM 91-0518.

Simulating Health Expenditures under Alternative Insurance Plans, 1993, free; RAND Corporation, order no. RP-205.

Trends in Hospital Average Lengths of Stay, Casemix, and Discharge Rates, 1980–1985, 1988; Agency for Health Care Policy and Research, order no. PHS 88-3420.

The Uninsured: How Many, 1992; Agency for Health Care Policy and Research, order no. 92-0101.

The Uninsured: Who Are They?, 1992; Agency for Health Care Policy and Research, order no. 92-0102.

Usual Sources of Medical Care and Their Characteristics, 1991; Agency for Health Care Policy and Research, order no. 91-0042.

Utilization and Costs in the CHAMPUS Reform Initiative: Preliminary Results for April–September 1989, 1991, $7.50; RAND Corporation, order no. N-3243-HA.

Utilization of Medical Services, 1993, $26.97; MGMA, order no. 4030.

Volume–Outcome Relationships and In-hospital Mortality: The Effect of Changes in Volume Over Time, 1992; Agency for Health Care Policy and Research, order no. 92-0046.

Health Insurance

Actuarial Issues in the Fee-For-Service/Prepaid Medical Group. 2nd edition, 1992; Medical Group Management Association.

Adolescent Health Insurance Status: Analyses of Trends in Coverage and Preliminary Estimates of the Effects of an Employer Mandate and Medicaid Expansion on the Uninsured, 1989; National Technical Information Service, order no. PB90-116-666.

AIDS and Health Insurance: An OTA Survey, 1988; National Technical Information Service, order no. PB88-170204.

Benefit Design in Health Care Reform: Clinical Preventive Service, 1993; Government Printing Office, stock no. 052-003-01340-1.

Benefit Design in Health Care Reform: Patient Cost-Sharing, 1993; Government Printing Office, stock no. 052-003-01339-8.

Characteristics of Health Insurance Coverage: Descriptive and Methodological Findings from the Health Insurance Experiment, 1986, $7.50; RAND Corporation, order no. N-2503-HHS.

Choices of Health Insurance and the Two-Worker Household, 1991; Agency for Health Care Policy and Research, order no. 91-0012.

Coverage of Preventative Services: Provisions of Selected Current Health Care Reform Proposals, 1993; National Technical Information Service, order no. PB94-126976.

Defense Health Care: Expansion of the CHAMPUS Reform Initiative into Washington and Oregon, 1993; General Accounting Office (HRD-93-149).

Defense Health Care: Lessons Learned From DOD's Managed Health Care Initiatives, 1993 Testimony, David P. Baine, Director, Federal Health Care Delivery Issues; General Accounting Office (T-HRD-93-21).

Does Health Insurance Make a Difference? 1992; National Technical Information Service, order no. PB93-101699.

Estimates of the Uninsured Population, Calendar Year 1987, 1990; Agency for Health Care Planning and Research, order no. PHS 90-3469.

Evaluation of the Oregon Medicaid Proposal Health Program, 1992; National Technical Information Service, order no. PB93-116192.

Expanding the Employer-Provided Health Insurance System: Effects on Workers and Their Employers, 1991, $16.50; The Urban Institute, ISBN no. 0-07766-509-5.

Health Insurance and the Demand for Medical Care: Evidence from a Randomized Experiment, 1988, $7.50; RAND Corporation, order no. R-3476-HHS.

Health Insurance: The Hawaii Experience, 1993; National Technical Information Service, order no. PB93-203743.

Health Insurance, Use of Health Services, and Health Care Expenditures, 1991; Agency for Health Care Planning and Research, order no. 92-0017.

The Impact of Being Uninsured on Utilization of Basic Health Care Services, 1992; Agency for Health Care Policy and Research, order no. 93-0030.

Insuring the Children: A Decade of Change, 1990; Agency for Health Care Policy and Research, order no. OM91-0519.

Medical Testing and Health Insurance, 1988; National Technical Information tion Service, order no. PB89-116958.

Multiple Sources of Medicare Supplementary Insurance, 1992; Agency for Health Care Policy and Research, order no. 92-0059.

1995–2000 Health Gain: Improving the Health of Communities through Integrated Healthcare, 1994, $85.00; HealthSpan.

1992–1995 Choice: America's Health Care Pluralism under Siege, 1994, $75.00; HealthSpan.

Private Health Insurance: Wide Variation in State Insurance Department's Regulatory Authority, Oversight, and Resources, 1993 Testimony, Leslie Aronovitz, Associate Director, Health Financing Issues; General Accounting Office (T-HRD-93-25).

Sharing the Burden—Strategies for Public and Private Long-Term Care Insurance, 1994, $34.95; The Brookings Institution, order no. 0-8157-9378-2.

Texas Health Care Reform: The Best and Worst Ideas, 1993, $10.00; National Center for Policy Analysis.

Twenty Myths about National Health Insurance, 1991, $10.00; National Center for Policy Analysis.

Two-Worker Families: Choice of Health Insurance, 1992; Agency for Health Care Planning and Research, order no. 92-0108.

Use of Medical Care in the RAND Health Insurance Experiment: Diagnosis and Service-Specific Analyses in a Randomized Controlled Trial, 1986, $10.00; RAND Corporation, order no. R-3469-HHS.

Hospital Management: General Management Information

America's Urban Health Safety Net: Preserving Access in the Era of Reform, 1991, $20.00; National Association of Public Hospitals.

Comparing Quality and Financial Performance of Accredited Hospitals, 1993; HCIA-JCAHO, order code JC-400.

Financially Distressed Hospitals: A Profile of Behavior before and after PPS, 1990; Agency for Health Care Policy and Research, order no. PHS 90-3467.

Health Care Access: Innovative Programs Using Nonphysicians, 1993; General Accounting Office (HRD-93-128).

Hospitals with Chronic Financial Losses: What Came Next, 1993; Agency for Health Care Policy and Research, order no. 93-0095.

Integrated Health Data Management Systems: A Tool for Avoiding Health Care Costs, 1990, $25.00; Washington Business Group on Health.

International Health Care Systems: A Chartbook Perspective, 2nd Edition, 1994, $30.00; AMA.

Managing Safety-Net Hospitals: Cases for Executive Development, 1993, $28.00; ACHE, order no. 0938.

1993 Salary and Benefits Report, USA, 1993, $50.00; Association for Healthcare Philanthropy.

1994 Outpatient Utilization Profile, 1994, $249.00; AMA.

Nonprofit Hospital: For-Profit Ventures Pose Access and Capacity Problems, 1993; General Accounting Office (HRD-93-124).

National Technical Information Service Alerts: Twice a month, the NTIS provides alerts, which are summaries of new data and titles added to the NTIS collection. Alerts are either prepackaged (on a number of topics such as *Healthcare and Computers*) or may be customized from a list of specified topics. Call (703) 487-4650 and ask for PR-797/CAU to receive a free catalogue describing the various topics. Prepackaged alerts vary in price from $135.00 to $250.00 per year (*Healthcare* is $135.00 per year). The price of customized alerts varies: one topic costs $100.00 per year, and additional topics cost $20.00 each. An annual index is available for some alerts (including *Healthcare*). The cost is $50.00.

National Technical Information Service Published Searches: National Technical Information Service Published Searches give full citations with abstracts on a specified topic, a subject index, and a title list of all articles found. Call (703) 487-4650 and ask for PR-186/CAU to receive a free copy of the *Published Search Master Catalogue, 1993* listing more than 2,000 searches.

Physician Supply and Utilization by Specialty: Trends and Projections, 1988, $40.00; AMA.

Putting the Pieces Together: A Guide to the Implementation of Integrated Health Data Management Systems, 1992, $45.00; Washington Business Group on Health.

State Health Care Data, 1993, $15.00; AMA.

The State of U.S. Hospitals in the Next Decade, 1989, $20.00; Association for Healthcare Philanthropy.

Strategic Alignment: Managing Integrated Health Systems, 1993; $34.00; ACHE, order no. 0937.

Hospital Management: Specific Hospital Service Lines

Cancer Services

Cancer Care and Cost: DRG's and Beyond, 1989, $28.00; ACHE, order no. 0895.

Children and Adolescent Services

Adolescent Health, Vol. 1: Summary and Policy Options, (H-468), 1991, 204 pages, $9.50; Government Printing Office, stock no. 052-003-01234-1.

Adolescent Health, Vol. 2: Background and the Effectiveness of Selected Prevention and Treatment Services, (H-466), 1991, 700 pages, $30.00; Government Printing Office, stock no. 52-003-01235-9.

Adolescent Health, Vol. 3: Crosscutting Issues in the Delivery of Health and Related Services, (H-467), 1991, 316 pages, $13.00; Government Printing Office, stock no. 052-003-01236-7.

Children as Capital: Corporate Health Policy Retreat, 1993; Washington Business Group on Health.

Children Without Health Insurance, 1992; Agency for Health Care Policy and Research, order no. 93-0025.

The Competitiveness and Productivity of Tomorrow's Workforce: Compelling Reasons for Investing in Healthy Children, 1993; Washington Business Group on Health.

The Effect of a Prepaid Group Practice on Children's Medical Care Use and Health Outcomes Compared to Fee-for-Service Care, 1989, $7.50; RAND Corporation, order no. N-2618-HHS.

The Effects of Cost Sharing on the Health of Children, 1986, $10.00; RAND Corporation, order no. R-3270-HHS.

Expenditures on Health Care for Children and Pregnant Women, 1992; Agency for Health Care Policy and Research, order no. 93-0022.

Healthy Children: Investing in the Future, 1988; National Technical Information Service, order no. PB88-178454.

Improving Access to Health Services for Children and Pregnant Women, 1991, $8.95; The Brookings Institution.

Incidence and Impact of Selected Infectious Diseases in Childhood, 1991; Government Printing Office, stock no. 017-022-01149-2, CDC.

Indian Adolescent Mental Health, 1990; National Technical Information Service, order no. PB90-254095.

Insuring the Children: A Decade of Change, 1990; Agency for Health Care Policy and Research, order no. OM91-0519.

Pediatric AIDS-Related Discharges in a Sample of U.S. Hospitals: Demographics, Diagnoses, and Resource Use, 1992; Agency for Health Care Policy and Research, order no. 92-0031.

Prepaid Group Practice Effects on the Utilization of Medical Services and Health Outcomes for Children: Results from a Controlled Trial, 1990, $4.00; RAND Corporation, order no. N-3116-HHS.

Preventive Health Care for Children: Experience from Selected Foreign Countries, 1993; General Accounting Office (HRD-93-62).

Technology Dependent Children: Hospital vs Home Care, 1987; National Technical Information Service, order no. PB87-194551.

Teen Pregnancy and Too-Early Childbearing, 1992, $8.00; Advocates for Youth.

Infectious Disease

AIDS in U.S. Hospitals, 1986–1987: A National Perspective, 1991; Agency for Health Care Policy and Research, order no. 91-0015.

Community-Based Care of Persons with AIDS: Developing a Research Agenda— AHCPR Conference Proceedings, 1990, 1991; Agency for Health Care Policy and Research, order no. PHS90-3456.

The Effectiveness of Drug Abuse Treatment: Implications for Controlling AIDS/HIV Infection, (PB-H-73), 1990; National Technical Information Service, order no. PB91-104885.

Forecasting the Medical Care Costs of the HIV Epidemic: 1991–1994, 1991; Agency for Health Care Planning and Research, order no. 92-0005.

Plagues, Products, and Politics—Emergent Public Health Hazards and National Policymaking, 1994, $34.95; The Brookings Institution, order no. 0-8157-2876-x.

U.S. General Population Projected AIDS Mortality Rates, 1989, 1989, $55.00; Society of Actuaries.

Mental Health

Children's Mental Health: Problems and Services, 1986; National Technical Information Service, order no. 3PB87-207486.

Criteria for Psychiatric Programs (Admission, Discharge, and Continued Stay Criteria), $15.00; National Association of Psychiatric Health Systems, item number CCP.

Defense Health Care: Additional Improvements Needed in CHAMPUS's Mental Health Program, 1993; General Accounting Office (HRD-93-34).

Defense Health Care: CHAMPUS Mental Health Demonstration Project in Virginia, 1992; General Accounting Office (HRD-93-53).

The Demand for Episodes of Mental Health Services, 1986, $20.00; RAND Corporation, order no. R-3432-NIMH.

Effects of Mental Health Insurance: Evidence from the Health Insurance Experiment, 1989, $4.00; RAND Corporation, order no. R-3815-NIMH-HCFA.

The Effects of Preferred Providers Options on Use of Outpatient Mental Health Services for Three Employee Groups, 1991, $7.50; RAND Corporation, order no. R-3952-HHS/NIMH.

Employee Assistance Programs: An Evolving Human Resource Management Strategy, 1992, $25.00; Washington Business Group on Health.

Mental Health, United States, 1992, 1992, $18.00; Government Printing Office, stock no. 017-024-01489-3.

1993 NAPHS Annual Survey: Final Report, $400.00; National Association of Psychiatric Health Systems.

Outcomes for Adult Outpatients with Depression under Prepaid or Fee-for-Service Financing, 1993, free; RAND Corporation, order no. RP-230.

Psychiatric Benefits in Employer-Provided Healthcare Plans: 1992 Report, $5.00; National Association of Psychiatric Health Systems, item no. HHR.

Psychiatric Fraud and Abuse: Increased Scrutiny of Hospital Stays Is Needed for Federal Health Programs, 1993; General Accounting Office (HRD-93-92).

Use of Outpatient Mental Health Care: Trial of a Prepaid Group Practice versus Fee-for-Service, 1986, $10.00; RAND Corporation, order no. R-3277-NIMH.

Utilization Review Survey, $20.00; National Association of Psychiatric Health Systems, item number URS.

Neuroscience and Rehabilitation

Charges and Outcomes for Rehabilitative Care: Implications for the Prospective Payment System, 1986, $7.50; RAND Corporation, order no. R-3424-HCFA.

Using Private Rehabilitation Vendors: Selection Criteria and Performance Standards to Ensure Quality, 1987, $20.00; Washington Business Group on Health.

Occupational Health

Biological Rhythms: Implications for the Worker, 1991; National Technical Information Service, order no. PB92-117589.

Cost Management in Employee Health Plans, 1987, $7.50; RAND Corporation, order no. R-3543-RWJ.

Employment-Related Health Insurance in 1987, 1993; Agency for Health Care Policy and Research, order no. 93-0044.

Health Benefits and the Workforce, 1992, $14.00; Government Printing Office, stock no. 029-000 00442-1.

Health Care Utilization in Employer Plans with Preferred Provider Organization Options, 1990, $7.50; RAND Corporation, order no. R-3800-HHS/NIMH.

Introducing the Preferred Provider Organization Option into Health Benefit Plans: Three Case Studies, 1990, $15.00; RAND Corporation, order no. N-2958-HHS.

Mandating Health Coverage for Working Americans, 1989; Agency for Health Care Policy and Research, order no. OM-90-0054.

Mandating Health Insurance Benefits for Employees: Effects on Health Care Use and Employers' Costs, 1989, $4.00; RAND Corporation, order no. N-2911-DOL.

Medical Monitoring and Screening in the Workplace: Results of a Survey, 1991, $4.50; Government Printing Office, stock no. 052-003-01255-3.

Occupation and Health Data Guide, Bibliographies and Data Sources from the National Center for Health Statistics, No. 2, 1993; CDC, order no. PHS 93-1308.

Participation and Satisfaction in Employer Plans with Preferred Provider Organization Options, 1990, $7.50; RAND Corporation, order no. R-3799-HHS/NIMH.

Primary Care

Annotated Bibliography of AHCPR Research on Non-physician Primary Care Providers, 1969–1989, 1990; Agency for Health Care Policy and Research, order no. OM 90-0073.

Health Care Reform, Primary Care, and the Need for Research, 1993; Agency for Health Care Policy and Research, order no. 93-0110.

Primary Care Research: An Agenda for the '90's, 1990; Agency for Health Care Policy and Research, order no. PHS 90-3460.

Primary Care Research: Theory and Methods. AHCPR Conference Proceedings, 1991; Agency for Health Care Policy and Research, order no. 91-0011.

A Research Agenda for Primary Care: Summary Report of a Conference, 1991; Agency for Health Care Policy and Research, order no. OM 91-0510.

Screening Mammography in Primary Care Settings: Implications for Cost, Access and Quality, 1991, National Technical Information Service, order no. PB92-182617.

Rural Health Care

Annotated Bibliography: Rural Health Services Research, 1968–90, 1991; Agency for Health Care Policy and Research, order no. 91-0014.

Defining Rural Areas: Impact on Health Care Policy and Research, 1989; National Technical Information Service, order no. PB89-224646.

Delivering Essential Health Care Services in Rural Areas: An Analysis of Alternative Models, 1991; Agency for Health Care Policy and Research, order no. 91-0017.

Health Care in Rural America, 1990; National Technical Information Service, order no. PB91-1-4927.

Rural Emergency Medical Services, 1989; National Technical Information Service, order no. PB90-159047.

Rural Health Care: The Future of the Hospital, 1990; Agency for Health Care Policy and Research, order no. OM 90-0055. *Rural Health Services: A Management Perspective,* 1994; ACHE, order no. 0948.

Rural and Urban Hospitals: Changes in Operations, Costs, and Revenues, 1981–1985, 1993; Agency for Health Care Policy and Research, order no. 93-0120.

Urban and Rural Hospital Costs: 1981–1985, 1988; Agency for Health Care Policy and Research, order no. PHS 88-3419.

Working from Within: Integrating Rural Health Care, 1993, $35.00; American Hospital Association, catalogue no. C-184151.

Senior Services

Aging America: Trends and Projections, 1993; Senate Committee on Aging.

Aging Issues: Related GAO Reports and Activities in Fiscal Year 1992, 1992; General Accounting Office (HRD-93-57).

Caring for the Disabled Elderly—Who Will Pay?, 1988, $36.95; The Brookings Institution, order no. 0-8157-7498-2.

Chartbook on Health Data on Older Americans: United States, 1992, $5.00; Government Printing Office, stock no. 017-022-00124-3, CDC.

Common Beliefs about the Rural Elderly: What Do National Data Tell Us? 1993, $5.00; Government Printing Office, stock no. 017-022-01205-7, CDC.

Eldercare in the Workplace: An Annotated Bibliography, 1994, $25.00; Washington Business Group on Health.

The Elderly with Functional Difficulties: Characteristics of Users of Home and Community Services, 1992; Agency for Health Care Policy and Research, order no. 92-0112.

The Elderly with Functional Difficulties: Patterns of Use of Home and Community Services, 1992; Agency for Health Care Policy and Research, order no. 92-0111.

Health Care after Retirement: Who Will Pay the Cost? 1989, $15.00; National Center for Policy Analysis.

Health Insurance Coverage of Retired Persons, 1989; National Technical Information Service, order no. PHS 89-3444.

Long-Term Care: Projected Needs of the Aging Baby Boom Generation, 1991; General Accounting Office (HRD-91-86).

Managing Health Care for Retirees: Employer Initiatives for the 1990's, 1994, $25.00; Washington Business Group on Health.

Nursing Home Residents: Demographic Characteristics and Functional Status, 1992; Agency for Health Care Policy and Research, order no. 92-0014.

Older Retirees: Supplements to Medicare Health Insurance Coverage, 1992; Agency for Health Care Policy and Research, order no. 92-0104.

Public/Private Partnerships in Health Promotion: A Guide for the Aging Network, 1994, $10.00; Washington Business Group on Health.

Retirees: Employment Related Health Insurance Coverage, 1992; Agency for Health Care Policy and Research, order no. 92-0103.

Retirees: Medicaid and Other Public Health Insurance Coverage, 1992; Agency for Health Care Policy and Research, order no. 92-0105.

Special Senate Committee on Aging Report, 1990; Senate Committee on Aging.

Women's Services

American Women's Health Care: A Patchwork Quilt with Gaps, 1992; Agency for Health Care Policy and Research, order no. 93-0008.

An Action Blueprint for Business: Forging New Partnerships to Make a Difference in Maternal and Child Health, 1993; Washington Business Group on Health.

The Corporate Perspective on Maternal and Child Health, 1989, $25.00; Washington Business Group on Health.

Cost Benefit Analysis of Preconception Care of Women with Established Diabetes Mellitus, 1993; Agency for Health Care Policy and Research, order no. 93-0100.

Economic Incentives in the Choice between Vaginal Delivery and Cesarean Section, 1994, free; RAND Corporation, order no. RP-246.

Improving Access to Health Services for Children and Pregnant Women, 1991, $8.95; The Brookings Institution.

Prenatal Care in the United States: A State and County Inventory (c. 1989), 1989, $50.00; The Alan Guttmacher Institute.

Managed Care

Adjusting Capitation Rates Using Objective Health Measures and Prior Utilization, 1989, $4.00; RAND Corporation, order no. N-2986-HCFA.

Capitation Utilization and Rate Guidebook, 1994, $995.00; St. Anthony Publishing.

Case-Mix Specialization in the Market for Hospital Services, 1990; Agency for Health Care Policy and Research, order no. OM 91-0521.

Clinical Classifications for Health Policy Research: Discharge Statistics by Principal Diagnosis and Procedure, 1993; Agency for Health Care Policy and Research, order no. 93-0043.

Compendium of State Systems for Resolutions of Medical Injury Claims, 1991; Agency for Health Care Planning and Research, order no. PHS 92-3474.

Consumer Acceptance of Prepaid and Fee-for-Service Medical Care: Results from a Randomized Controlled Trial, 1986, $4.00; RAND Corporation, order no. N-2692-HHS.

A Controlled Trial of the Effect of a Prepaid Group Practice on the Utilization of Medical Services, 1985, $4.00; RAND Corporation, order no. R-3029-HHS.

Creating New Health Care Ventures: The Role of Management, 1991, $73.00; Aspen Publishers.

Health Care CBA/CEA: An Update on the Growth and Composition of the Literature, 1993; Agency for Health Care Policy and Research, order no. 93-0101.

Health Care: Rochester's Community Approach Yields Better Access, Lower Costs, 1993; General Accounting Office (HRD-93-44).

HMO Market Share and Its Effect on Local Medicare Costs, 1991, $8.50; The Urban Institute.

Impact of AIDS on the Kaiser Permanente Medical Care Program (Northern California Region), 1988; National Technical Information Service, order no. PB89-116941.

Inequities in Hospital Care: The Massachusetts Experiment, 1991; Agency for Health Care Policy and Research, order no. 92-0006.

Integrated Health Care: Case Studies, 1993, $35.00; MGMA, order no. 4066.

Integrated Health Care: Reorganizing the Physician, Hospital and Health Plan Relationship, 1993, $48.00; MGMA, order no. 4065.

Integration Issues in Physician/Hospital Affiliations, 1993, $49.00; MGMA, order no. 3912.

Joint Ventures between Hospitals and Physicians: A Competitive Strategy for the Healthcare Marketplace, 1987, $59.00; Aspen Publishers.

Making Managed Care Work: A Practical Guide to Strategies and Solutions, 1992, $84.00; Aspen Publishers.

Managed Care Contracts Manual, 1994, $225.00; Aspen Publishers.

Managed Care Law Manual, 1994, $229.00; Aspen Publishers.

Managed Care Quarterly, $94.00; Aspen Publishers.

The Managed Health Care Handbook, Second Edition, 1993, $94.00; Aspen Publishers.

Medicaid: States Turn to Managed Care to Improve Access and Control Costs, 1993; General Accounting Office (HRD-99-46).

Meeting the Health Care Crisis, 1991, $20.00; National Association of Manufacturers.

The New Healthcare Market: A Guide to PPOs for Purchasers, Payors, and Providers, 1988, $95.00; Aspen Publishers.

1991–1996 The Trauma of Transformation in the 1990's, 1994, $75.00; Deloitte & Touche/HealthSpan.

The Physician's Guide to Managed Care, 1993; Aspen Publishers.

Physician–Hospital Alliances: Strategies for Building Quality Health Care Systems, 1994, $149.00; Aspen Publishers.

Preferred Provider Organizations: Planning, Structure, and Operation, 1984, $68.00; Aspen Publishers.

A Primer on Managed Competition, 1994, $10.00; National Center for Policy Analysis.

Transforming the Delivery of Health Care: Mergers, Acquisitions, and Physician–Hospital Organizations, 1992, $85.00; MGMA, order no. 3303.

Physician Supply

Note: For statistical data on physician issues, see the subheading Physician Issues under the main heading Statistical Data and Surveys (Compilations).

Creating New Hospital–Physician Collaboration, 1993, $37.00; ACHE, order no. 0931.

Effective Hospital–Physician Relationships, 1990, $33.00; ACHE, order no. 0900.

High-Cost Medical Staffs: A Policy Option for Controlling the Volume of Physician Services in the Hospital, 1992, $11.00; The Urban Institute, working paper no. 3982-04.

How Do Medicare Physician Fees Compare to Private Payers? 1993, $8.50; The Urban Institute, working paper no. 6197.

Paying Physicians: Options for Controlling Cost, Volume, and Intensity of Services, 1992, $30.00; ACHE, order no. 0920.

Physician Bonding, 1989, $55.00; Aspen Publishers.

Physicians and Management in Health Care, 1992, $36.00; Aspen Publishers.

Salaries and Fringe Benefits—HMO Physicians, 1993, $10.00; MGMA, order no. 3622.

Salaries and Fringe Benefits—Physicians (Fringe Benefits), 1993, $43.77; MGMA, order no. 3538.

Salaries and Fringe Benefits—Physicians (Time Off Allowances), 1993, $35.94; MGMA, order no. 3649.

Statistical Data and Surveys (Compilations)

Note: For statistics on utilization, see the subheading Utilization Reports and Statistical Summaries under the main heading Health Care Utilization.

General References

AHA Hospital Statistics, 1994, $139.00; AHA, catalog no. C-082094.

A Compilation of Analyses of Economic Impacts of Competing Approaches to Health Care Reform by Experts and Stakeholders, 1993, $8.00; Government Printing Office, stock no. 052-003-01327.

The DRG Handbook: Comparative Clinical and Financial Standards (Medicare data), 1994, $399.00 (paper), $1,299.00 (diskette); Health Care Investment Analysts.

Health United States 1992 and Healthy People 2000 Review, 1993, $30.00; Government Printing Office, stock no. 017-022-01218-9.

Healthy People 2000: National Health Promotion and Disease Prevention Objectives, 1991, $9.00; Government Printing Office, stock no. 017-001-00473-1.

International Health Statistics: What the Numbers Mean for the United States, 1993, $11.00; Government Printing Office, stock no. 052-003-01354-1.

Mental Health, United States, 1992, 1992, $18.00; Government Printing Office, stock no. 017-024-01489-3.

The National Hospital Panel Survey Reports, monthly reports, call for price; AHA, catalog no. C-084194.

1990 Census of Population and Housing-Parts A & B, 1992–93, Part A, $11.00 (Government Printing Office, stock no. 003-024-08574-7), Part B, $5.50 (Government Printing Office, stock no. 003-024-08679-4).

The Outpatient Utilization Profile, (Medicare Data), 1994, $249.00 (paper), $899.00 (diskette); Health Care Investment Analysts.

Population Profile of the United States, 1993, 1993, $8.50; Government Printing Office, stock no. 803-005-10038-3.

State-Level Data Book on Health Care Access and Financing, 1993, $35.00; The Urban Institute, ISBN no. 0-87766-597-4.

Health Insurance and Managed Care

Note: Nonstatistical information on these topics can be found under the main headings Health Insurance and Managed Care as well as under the subheadings under the heading Directories and Basic Reference Books.

Mid-Sized Employer Health Plans, 1993, 1994, $100.00; A. Foster Higgins.

National Survey of Employer-Sponsored Health Plans—1993, 1994, $500.00; A. Foster Higgins.

1994 Annual Survey of State Employee Health Benefit Plans, 1994; Medical Software Products.

Preferred Provider Organizations: Industry Characteristics, Growth, and Trends, 1991, 1991, $100.00; American Association of Preferred Provider Organizations.

Report and Tables (from National Survey of Employer-Sponsored Health Plans-1993), 1994, $100.00; A. Foster Higgins.

Source Book of Health Insurance Data, $12.00; HIAA.

Statistical Compilation—Life/Health, 1992, $150.00; National Association of Insurance Commissioners, order no. STA-LS.

Trends in Health Benefits, 1993, $13.00; Government Printing Office, stock no. 029-000-00445-5.

Utilization of Medical Services, 1993, $26.97; MGMA, order no. 4030.

Length of Stay

LOS by Diagnosis and Operation, 1994, $164.00; AMA.

Length of Stay by Diagnosis and Operation—North Central (Northeastern, Southern, Western), 1994, $164.00 per region, complete five-volume set $659.00; Health Care Investment Analysts.

National Length of Stay by Diagnosis and Operation, 1994, $164.00 (paper), call for electronic media price; Health Care Investment Analysts.

National Length of Stay by DRG and Payment Source, 1994, $164.00; Health Care Investment Analysts.

National Psychiatric Length of Stay by Diagnosis and Operation, 1994, $110.00; Health Care Investment Analysts.

Psychiatric Length of Stay by Diagnosis and Operation—Northeastern (North Central, Southern, Western), 1994, $110.00 per region; Health Care Investment Analysts.

Physician Issues

Medical Groups in the U.S. 1993, 1994, $70.00; AMA.

Physician Characteristics and Distribution in the U.S. 1994, 1994, $95.00; AMA.

Physician Data by County 1993, 1994, $159.00; AMA.

Physician Marketplace Statistics 1993, 1994, $225.00; AMA.

Physicians in Medical Groups: A Comparative Analysis 1993, 1994, $95.00; AMA.

Practice Patterns of General Internal Medicine—First Edition, 1994, $50.00; AMA.

Socioeconomic Characteristics of Medical Practice 1994, 1994, $165.00; AMA.

Quality and Financial Performance

Administrative Costs in Healthcare: U.S. and Canada, 1994; Office of Technology Assessment.

The Comparative Performance of U.S. Hospitals: The Source Book, 1994, $439.00 (paper), $1,299.00 (diskette); Health Care Investment Analysts.

Comparing Quality and Financial Performance of Accredited Hospitals, 1994, $95.00; Health Care Investment Analysts.

Cross-national Study of Hospital Spending, 1994; Office of Technology Assessment.

HCIA Guide to Hospital Performance, 1993, 1994, $995.00; AMA.

Hospital Accreditation Statistics, 1986–88, 1988, $50.00; JCAHO.

The 1994 National Executive Poll on Health Care Costs and Benefits, 1994, $24.95; Business and Health.

Publications from the 1987 National Medical Expenditure Survey NMES II, 1993; Agency for Health Care Policy and Research, order no. 93-0035.

Information for Ordering Studies and Reports

This section contains the sources for the preceding reports, including addresses and phone and fax numbers. In addition, this section includes additional organizations, addresses, and phone and fax numbers that may be useful to readers.

A. Foster Higgins

A. Foster Higgins
125 Broad Street
New York, NY 10004
(212) 574-9025 phone

ACHE

The Foundation of the American College of Healthcare Executives
Order Processing Center, Dept. 93
1951 Cornell Avenue
Melrose Park, IL 60160-1001
(312) 424-2800 phone

Advance Data

Single copies of the Advance Data reports may be obtained free of charge by writing the National Center for Health Statistics, Scientific and Technical Information Branch, 6525 Belcrest Road, Hyattsville, MD 20872. Specify the Advance Data report number you wish to receive.

Advocates for Youth (formerly The Center for Population Options)

Advocates for Youth
1025 Vermont Avenue, N.W., Suite 200
Washington, DC 20005
(202) 347-5700 phone
(202) 347-2263 fax

Agency for Health Care Policy and Research

U.S. Department of Health and Human Services
Public Health Service
Agency for Health Care Policy and Research
Executive Office Center, Suite 501
2101 East Jefferson Street
Rockville, MD 20852

AHA

The American Hospital Association publishes an extensive collection of resource materials. Mail, telephone, or fax orders by catalog number to:

AHA Services, Inc.
P.O. Box 92683
Chicago, IL 60675-2683
(800) AHA-2626 phone
(312) 422-4505 fax

MasterCard, VISA, American Express, or institutional/company purchase order number are accepted. A company purchase order is required for billed orders. Personal orders must be accompanied by a check or credit card information. Members of the American Hospital Association receive a discount on materials.

In addition to its publications *AHA Guide to the Health Care Field*, *AHA Hospital Statistics*, and *Economic Trends*, AHA's Health Statistics Group offers a number of other products that may be of interest to health care managers and planners. These include:

AHA Abridged Guide to the Health Care Field on Diskette
National Hospital Panel Survey Reports
AHA Annual Survey Database on Tape
AHA MRI Utilization Model

Questions about these publications and products can be directed to:

Health Statistics Group
American Hospital Association
One North Franklin
Chicago, IL 60606
(312) 422-3990 phone
(312) 422-4570 fax
(800) AHA-2626 (to place an order)

A further data resource at the American Hospital Association is the AHA Resource Center. Drawing on its collection of over 55,000 volumes on health care administration, the Resource Center can provide access to information about most printed data sources:

American Hospital Association
AHA Resource Center
One North Franklin
Chicago, IL 60606
(312) 422-2000 phone
(312) 422-4700 fax

Alan Guttmacher Institute

The Alan Guttmacher Institute
120 Wall Street, Suite 21
New York, NY 10005
(212) 248-1111 phone
(212) 248-1951 fax

All orders must be prepaid in U.S. currency by check, VISA, or MasterCard.

Allina Health System/Deloitte & Touche

Allina Health System/Deloitte & Touche
Attention: Editor, Environmental Assessment
2810 Fifty-Seventh Avenue North
Minneapolis, MN 55430
(612) 574-7618 phone

AMA

American Medical Association
Attention: Order Department
P.O. Box 7046
Dover, DE 19903
(800) 621-8335 phone

Payment by check or credit card (VISA, MasterCard, or American Express) must accompany all orders.

American Association of Preferred Provider Organizations

American Association of Preferred Provider Organizations
601 13th Street N.W., Suite 370
Washington, DC 20005
(202) 347-7600 phone
(202) 347-7601 fax

Aspen Publishers, Inc.

Aspen Publishers, Inc.
7201 McKinney Circle
P.O. Box 990
Frederick, MD 21701-9782
(800) 638-8437 phone
(301) 693-7931 fax

Association for the Advancement of Health Education

Association for the Advancement of Health Education
1900 Association Drive
Reston, VA 22091
(703) 476-3437 phone
(703) 476-9527 fax

Association for Healthcare Philanthropy

Association for Healthcare Philanthropy
313 Park Avenue, Suite 400
Falls Church, VA 22046
(703) 532-6243 phone
(703) 532-7170 fax

All orders must be prepaid by check, money order, or credit card in U.S.
funds.

The Brookings Institution

The Brookings Institution
Book Order Department
P.O. Box 029
Washington, DC 20042-0029
(800) 275-1447 phone
(202) 797-6004 fax

BRS Information Technologies

BRS Information Technologies
A Division of InfoPro Technologies, Inc.
8000 Westpark Drive
McLean, VA 22102
(800) 289-4377 phone
(800) 456-7248 phone
(703) 442-0900 phone in VA

Bureau of Labor Statistics

Bureau of Labor Statistics
Publication Sales Center
P.O. Box 2145
Chicago, IL 60690
(312) 353-1880 (phone)

Business and Health

Business and Health
5 Paragon Drive
Montvale, NJ 07645
(201) 358-7300 phone

CISTI

Canada Institute for Scientific & Technical Information
National Research Council Canada
Ottawa, Ontario K1A 0S2
Canada
(613) 993-1210 phone
(613) 952-8244 fax

Catholic Health Association

Catholic Health Association
1776 K Street, N.W., Suite 204
Washington, DC 20006
(202) 296-3993 phone
(202) 296-3997 fax

CDC

U.S. Department of Health & Human Services
Public Health Service
Centers for Disease Control and Prevention
National Center for Health Statistics
6525 Belcrest Road
Hyattsville, MD 20872

CDP Online Services

CDP Technologies, Inc.
333 7th Avenue
New York, NY 10001
(800) 289-4277 phone
(212) 563-3784 fax

Children of Alcoholics Foundation

Children of Alcoholics Foundation
P.O. Box 4185, Grand Central Station
New York, NY 10163-4185
(212) 754-0656 phone
(212) 754-0664 fax

Citizen Action

Citizen Action
1730 Rhode Island Avenue, N.W., Suite 403
Washington, DC 20036
(202) 775-1580 phone

Congressional Budget Office

Congressional Budget Office
Ford House Office Building
2nd and D Streets, S.W.
Washington, DC 20515
(202) 226-2621 phone

Deloitte & Touche/HealthSpan

Deloitte & Touche/HealthSpan
125 Summer Street
Boston, MA 02110
(617) 737-7570 phone

DIALOG DATA-STAR

DIALOG DATA-STAR
1 Commerce Square
2005 Market Street, Suite 1010
Philadelphia, PA 19103
(800) 221-7754 phone
(215) 687-6777 phone in PA

DIALOG Information Services

DIALOG Information Services
3460 Hillview Avenue
Palo Alto, CA 94304
(800) 334-2564 phone

European Space Agency/Research Institute

European Space Agency/Research Institute
P.O. Box 64
Via Galileo Galilei
00044 Frascati (Rome), Italy
11-39/6 94180361 fax

General Accounting Office

U.S. General Accounting Office
Office of Information Management and Communications
Document Distribution Center
P.O. Box 6015
Gaithersburg, MD 20884-6015
(202) 512-6000 phone
(301) 258-4066 fax

The first copy of each report and testimony is free. Additional copies are $2.00 each. Orders must be prepaid in cash or by check or money order made out to the Superintendent of Documents. There is a 25 percent discount on orders for 100 or more copies mailed to a single address.

Government Printing Office

U.S. Government Printing Office
Superintendent of Documents
P.O. Box 371954
Pittsburgh, PA 15250-7954
(202) 512-1800 phone
(202) 512-2250 fax

Orders must include the title, Government Printing Office stock number, quantity, price, and total payment. Orders may be paid for by check, VISA, MasterCard, GPO Deposit Account, or money order. If using VISA or MasterCard, the card number and expiration date must be included. The Government Printing Office pays normal shipping; however, it will arrange and bill the recipient for United Parcel Service and first-class and airmail services. Call (202) 512-1800 in advance to determine rates and arrange for this service.

Orders may be sent by facsimile; machines are available 24 hours a day, seven days a week. When using fax services, orders must be paid for using VISA or MasterCard.

Group Health Association of America

Group Health Association of America
1129 Twentieth Street, N.W., Suite 600
Washington, DC 20036
(202) 778-3200 phone

Prepayment is required. Phone orders are accepted with an American Express card.

HCFA

Health Care Financing Administration
East Highrise Building
FOHR/Publications
6325 Security Boulevard
Baltimore, MD 21207-5187
(410) 966-7843 phone

HCFA publications are ordered through the NTIS (see address and ordering information in this section).

Health Care Investment Analysts

Health Care Investment Analysts
300 East Lombard Street
Baltimore, MD 21202
(800) 568-3282 phone
(410) 539-5220 fax

Health Care Investment Analysts
P.O. Box 303
Ann Arbor, MI 48106-0303
(800) 521-6210 phone

Health Resources and Services Administration, Bureau of Health Professions, Office of Research and Planning

Health Resources and Services Administration, Bureau of Health
   Professions, Office of Research and Planning
Room 8-47, Parklawn Building
5600 Fishers Lane
Rockville, MD 20857
(301) 443-6936 phone
(301) 443-8003 fax

Health Resources and Services Administration,
Bureau of Health Resources Development, Division of HIV Services

Health Resources and Services Administration, Bureau of Health
  Resources Development, Division of HIV Services
Room 7a-55, Parklawn Building
5600 Fishers Lane
Rockville, MD 20857
(301) 443-6745 phone
(301) 443-5271 fax

Health Resources and Services Administration,
Bureau of Primary Health Care, Division of Federal Occupational Health

Health Resources and Services Administration,
Bureau of Primary Health Care, Division of Federal
Occupational Health
4350 East-West Highway, Room 32A2
Bethesda, MD 20814
(301) 594-0250 phone
(301) 594-4991 fax

Health Resources and Services Administration,
Bureau of Primary Health Care, National Clearinghouse for Primary
Care Information

Health Resources and Services Administration, Bureau of Primary
  Health Care, National Clearinghouse for Primary Care Information
8201 Greensboro Drive, Suite 600
McLean, VA 22102
(703) 821-8955, ext. 248 phone
(703) 821-2098 fax

Health Resources and Services Administration,
Bureau of Primary Health Care, National Maternal and Child Health
Clearinghouse

Health Resources and Services Administration, Bureau of Primary
  Health Care, National Maternal and Child Health Clearinghouse
8201 Greensboro Drive, Suite 600
McLean, VA 22102
(703) 821-8955, ext. 254 phone
(703) 821-2098 fax

HIAA

Health Insurance Association of America
1025 Connecticut Avenue, N.W., Suite 1200
Washington, DC 20036-3998
(202) 223-7780 phone
(202) 223-7896 fax

Hewitt Associates

Hewitt Associates
100 Half Day Road
Lincolnshire, IL 60069
(708) 295-5000 phone

Institute for Alternative Futures

Institute for Alternative Futures
100 North Pitt Street
Alexandria, VA 22314
(703) 684-5880 phone
(703) 684-0640 fax

InterStudy Publications

InterStudy Publications
c/o Decision Resources, Inc.
Bay Colony Corporate Center
110 Winter Street
Waltham, MA 02154-9916
(617) 487-3700 phone
(617) 487-5750 fax

JCAHO

Joint Commission on Accreditation of Healthcare Organizations
P.O. Box 75751
Chicago, IL 60675-5751
(708) 916-5800 phone

All mail orders must be prepaid in U.S. funds. Discounts are available
for orders of 16–50 copies of the same publication (10 percent), 51–100
copies of the same publication (15 percent), and 101–500 copies of the
same publication (20 percent). VISA and MasterCard orders will be
accepted by phone or fax.

KMPG Peat Marwick

KMPG Peat Marwick
P.O. Box 23331
Newark, NJ 07189
(201) 467-9650 phone

Knowledge Express

Knowledge Express
900 West Valley Road
Suite 401
Wayne, PA 19087
(800) 248-2469 phone

Marion Merrell Dow

Marion Merrell Dow, Inc.
P.O. Box 8410
Kansas City, MO 64114
(800) 821-4703 phone
(816) 966-4000 phone
(816) 966-3820 fax

Medical Software Products

Medical Software Products
591 West Hamilton Avenue, Suite 205
Campbell, CA 95008
(408) 370-9440 phone
(800) 444-4570 phone
(408) 370-3393 fax

MGMA

Medical Group Management Association
104 Inverness Terrace East
Englewood, CO 80112-5306
(303) 643-4422 phone
(303) 643-4427 fax
(303) 643-4422 automatic phone ordering system (credit card required
if not a member)

Prepayment is required if not a member. Phone orders can be taken with
VISA, MasterCard, or American Express. Prices quoted are for non-
members; MGMA members and affiliates receive significant discounts.

Midwest Business Group on Health

Midwest Business Group on Health
8303 West Higgins Road, Suite 200
Chicago, IL 60631
(312) 380-9090 phone

Milliman & Robertson

Milliman & Robertson, Inc.
Actuaries and Consultants
1301 Fifth Avenue, Suite 3800
Seattle, WA 98101-2605
(206) 624-7940 phone
(206) 340-1380 fax

NAHDO

National Association of Health Data Organizations
254-B North Washington Street
Falls Church, VA 22046-4517
(703) 532-3282 phone
(703) 532-3593 fax

National Association of Insurance Commissioners

National Association of Insurance Commissioners
120 West 12th Street, Suite 1100
Kansas City, MO 64105-1925
(816) 374-7259 phone
(816) 471-7004 fax

National Association of Manufacturers

National Association of Manufacturers
1331 Pennsylvania Avenue, N.W., Suite 1500
Washington, DC 20004-1703
(202) 367-3086 phone
(800) 637-3005 phone
(202) 637-3182 fax

All orders must be prepaid by check or credit card (VISA, MasterCard, American Express).

National Association of Psychiatric Health Systems

National Association of Psychiatric Health Systems
1319 F Street, N.W., Suite 1000
Washington, DC 20004
(202) 393-6700 phone
(202) 783-6041 fax

National Association of Public Hospitals

National Association of Public Hospitals
1212 New York Avenue, N.W., Suite 800
Washington, DC 20005
(202) 408-0223 phone
(202) 408-0235 fax

National Business Coalition on Health

National Business Coalition on Health
1015 18th Street, N.W., Suite 450
Washington, DC 20036
(202) 775-9300 phone

National Center for Policy Analysis

National Center for Policy Analysis
12655 North Central Expressway, Suite 720
Dallas, TX 75243-1739
(214) 386-6272 phone
(214) 386-0924 fax

National Health Council

National Health Council
350 Fifth Avenue, Suite 1118
New York, NY 10118

National Technical Information Service

National Technical Information Service
5285 Port Royal Road
Springfield, VA 22161
(703) 487-4650 phone
(703) 321-8547 fax
(703) 487-4815 fax

NERAC, Inc.

NERAC, Inc.
One Technology Drive
Tolland, CT 06084-9919
(203) 872-7000 phone

NLM

National Library of Medicine
8600 Rockville Pike
Bethesda, MD 20894
(800) 638-8480 phone
(301) 496-6193 phone

Northwestern National Life Insurance Companies

Northwestern National Life Insurance Companies
P.O. Box 20, Route 6528
Minneapolis, MN 55440
(612) 342-7137 phone
(612) 372-1015 fax

The first copy of a document is free; others are $5.00 each.

Office of National Health Statistics

Office of National Health Statistics
Attention: Ross Arnett
HealthCare Financing Administration
L-1, EQ 05, 6235 Security Boulevard
Baltimore, MD 21207
(410) 966-7933 phone

Office of Technology Assessment

Publications Order
U.S. Congress Office of Technology Assessment
Washington, DC 20510-8025
(202) 224-8996 phone
(202) 228-6098 fax

ORBIT/QUESTEL, Inc.

ORBIT/QUESTEL, Inc.
8000 Westpark Drive
McLean, VA 22102
(800) 456-7248 phone
(703) 442-0900 phone in VA

The Pace Group

The Pace Group
12160 Abrams Road, Suite 409
Dallas, TX 75243
(214) 437-5611 phone

The Prevention Index

The Prevention Index
33 East Minor Street
Emmaus, PA 18098
(215) 967-5171 phone

RAND Corporation

RAND Corporation
Attention: Distribution Services
1700 Main Street
P.O. Box 2138
Santa Monica, CA 90407-2138
(310) 451-7002 phone
(310) 451-6915 fax
order@rand.org e-mail via Internet

Orders must be prepaid with check, money order, or credit card (VISA, MasterCard).

Robert Wood Johnson Foundation

Robert Wood Johnson Foundation
College Road, P.O. Box 2316
Princeton, NJ 08543-2316
(609) 243-5929 phone

St. Anthony Publishing, Inc.

St. Anthony Publishing, Inc.
P.O. Box 96561
Washington, DC 20090-6561
(800) 632-0123 phone
(703) 707-5700 fax

Segal Company

Segal Company
1 Park Avenue
New York, NY 10016
(212) 251-5059 phone
(212) 251-5490 fax

Self-Insurance Institute of America

Self-Insurance Institute of America
P.O. Box 15466
Santa Ana, CA 92705
(714) 261-2553 phone

Senate Committee on Aging

Senate Committee on Aging
Attention: Publications
G-31 Dirksen Building
Washington, DC 20510
(202) 224-5364 phone

SilverPlatter Information, Inc.

SilverPlatter Information, Inc.
100 River Ridge Drive
Norwood, MA 02062
(800) 343-0064 phone

SMG Marketing Group, Inc.

SMG Marketing Group, Inc.
1342 North LaSalle Street
Chicago, IL 60610
(312) 642-3026 phone
(312) 642-9729 fax

Society of Actuaries

Society of Actuaries
Research Department
475 North Martingale Road, Suite 800
Schaumburg, IL 60173
(708) 706-3500 phone
(708) 706-3599 fax

STN International

STN International
2540 Olentangy River Road
P.O. Box 3012
Columbus, OH 43210
(800) 848-6533 phone
(800) 848-6538 phone in OH and Canada

The Urban Institute

UPA Order Department
c/o The Urban Institute
4720 Boston Way
Lanham, MD 20706
(800) 462-6420 phone
(301) 459-2118 fax

All orders by individuals must be prepaid by check, VISA, or MasterCard.

U.S. Chamber of Commerce

U.S. Chamber of Commerce
Publications Fulfillment
1615 H Street, N.W.
Washington, DC 20062
(800) 638-6582 phone

U.S. House of Representatives

U.S. House of Representatives
U.S. House Documents Room
Washington, DC 20515
(202) 224-3121 phone

Washington Business Group on Health

Washington Business Group on Health
Attention: Publications
777 North Capitol Street NE, Suite 800
Washington, DC 20002
(202) 408-9320 phone
(202) 408-9332 fax

Williams & Wilkins

Williams & Wilkins
P.O. Box 1496
Baltimore, MD 21298-9724
(800) 638-0672 phone

Additional Books of Interest

Benchmarking in Health Care: A Collaborative Approach

by Robert G. Gift and Doug Mosel

This book, with a two-part foreword by Robert C. Camp, Ph.D., and Philip A. Newbold, presents a novel four-phase collaborative approach to performing benchmarking studies. Readers receive guidance on how to collaborate with other health care organizations to conduct studies that examine and compare business and clinical practices. This collaborative approach to benchmarking can be used as a tool for continuous quality improvement. Benchmarking can help health care providers move beyond the incremental improvements associated with quality improvement to quick, dramatic performance improvement in key processes.

Catalog No. E99-169107 (must be included when ordering)
1994. 212 pages, 72 figures.
$49.00 (AHA members, $39.00)

The Health Care Organizational Survey System

by Donald N. Lombardi, Ph.D.

This book helps you gather data in support of your TQM efforts by starting a survey program in your institution or modifying your existing survey to make it more effective. Included are field-tested survey questions, a series of supplemental survey items that can be used to customize the survey instrument, and a handbook for conducting a "do-it-yourself" survey. The Survey Analysis Guides present response indicators for questions in the survey and help you interpret the response, and the action plans can be tailored to the organization, department, or individual level.

Catalog No. E99-088175 (must be included when ordering)
1994. 200 pages, 18 figures, 4 appendixes.
$50.00 (AHA members, $40.00)

To order, call TOLL FREE 1-800-AHA-2626